# Greatest
# Kan and Li

## Gathering
## the Cosmic Light

Mantak Chia
and Andrew Jan

Destiny Books
Rochester, Vermont • Toronto, Canada

Destiny Books
One Park Street
Rochester, Vermont 05767
www.DestinyBooks.com

Destiny Books is a division of Inner Traditions International

Originally published in Thailand in 2012 by Universal Tao Publications

**Library of Congress Cataloging-in-Publication Data**
Chia, Mantak, 1944– author.
  Greatest Kan and Li : gathering the cosmic light / Mantak Chia and Andrew Jan.
    pages cm
  Originally published: Thailand : Universal Tao Publications, 2012.
  Summary: "A fully illustrated guide to the most advanced Kan and Li practice to birth the immortal spirit body and unite with the Tao" — Provided by publisher.
  Includes bibliographical references and index.
  ISBN 978-1-62055-231-5 (paperback) — ISBN 978-1-62055-232-2 (e-book)
  1. Taoism. 2. Spiritual healing. I. Jan, Andrew, author. II. Title.
  BL1923.C44 2014
  299.5'1444—dc23
                                                                2013049631

Printed and bound in the United States by Versa Press, Inc.

10  9  8  7  6  5  4  3  2  1

Text design by Priscilla Baker and layout by Virginia Scott Bowman
This book was typeset in Garamond Premier Pro and Futura with Diotima, Present, Sho, and Gill Sans used as display typefaces

Illustrations by Udon Jandee
Photographs by Sopitnapa Promnon

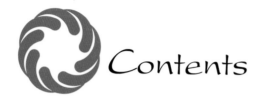

# Contents

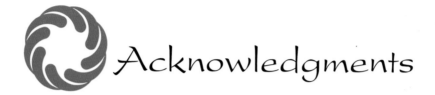

# Acknowledgments

The Universal Tao publications staff involved in the preparation and production of *Greatest Kan and Li: Gathering the Cosmic Light* extend our gratitude to the many generations of Taoist Masters who have passed on their special lineage, in the form of an unbroken oral transmission, over thousands of years. We thank Taoist Master I Yun (Yi Eng) for his openness in transmitting the formulas of Taoist Inner Alchemy.

We offer our eternal gratitude to our parents and teachers for their many gifts to us. Remembering them brings joy and satisfaction to our continued efforts in presenting the Universal Healing Tao system. For their gifts, we offer our eternal gratitude and love. As always, their contribution has been crucial in presenting the concepts and techniques of the Universal Healing Tao.

We wish to thank the thousands of unknown men and women of the Inner Alchemy arts who developed many of the methods and ideas presented in this book. Beyond the Taoist community we would like to devote this text to all the meditative (mystical) traditions of the world. There is a commonality in all religions and it is my hope that such texts as this one can benefit all those who study Inner Alchemy. Taoism has early roots in Hindu mystical practice with an ongoing cross-pollination with Buddhism over recent millennia. Many of the Western alchemical traditions are likely to have originated in the East. Furthermore, we thank one successful immortal for shaping our early spiritual lives. His name is, of course, Jesus Christ.

We wish to thank Colin Drown for his editorial work.

We thank the many contributors essential to this book's final form: the editorial and production staff at Inner Traditions/Destiny Books for their efforts to clarify the text and produce a handsome new edition of the book, and Gail Rex for her line edit of the new edition.

For their efforts on the first edition of this book, we thank our Thai production team: Hirunyathorn Punsan, Sopitnapa Promnon, Udon Jandee, and Suthisa Chaisarn.

# Putting the Greatest Kan and Li Meditation into Practice

The practices described in this book have been used successfully for thousands of years by Taoists trained by personal instruction. Readers should not undertake the practice without receiving personal transmission and training from a certified instructor of the Universal Healing Tao, since certain of these practices, if done improperly, may cause injury or result in health problems. This book is intended to supplement individual training by the Universal Healing Tao and to serve as a reference guide for these practices. Anyone who undertakes these practices on the basis of this book alone does so entirely at his or her own risk.

The meditations, practices, and techniques described herein are not intended to be used as an alternative or substitute for professional medical treatment and care. If any readers are suffering from illnesses based on mental or emotional disorders, an appropriate professional health care practitioner or therapist should be consulted. Such problems should be corrected before you start training.

Neither the Universal Healing Tao nor its staff and instructors can be responsible for the consequences of any practice or misuse of the information contained in this book. If the reader undertakes any exercise without strictly following the instructions, notes, and warnings, the responsibility must lie solely with the reader.

With specific reference to the chapter on diet: the authors strongly advise against self-medicating with herbs or fasting unsupervised. Herbs should only be taken under the direct supervision of a qualified herbal practitioner. Likewise partial fasting and complete fasting should also be carried out under medical supervision.

This book does not attempt to give any medical diagnosis, treatment, prescription, or remedial recommendation in relation to any human disease, ailment, suffering, or physical condition whatsoever.

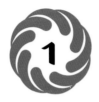

# Taoist History Related to the Greatest Kan and Li Meditation

*At the moment of that cry [birth of the spiritual infant],\**
*the conscious spirit of the generations of history also*
*enters into the opening and merges with the primordial*
*original spirit.*

LIU I-MING[1]

This chapter continues the discussion we began in *The Practice of Greater Kan and Li* about the historical context of the Universal Healing Tao (UHT) Kan and Li practice among the other Taoist schools.†

There are many practices or gates to the Tao, of which the Kan and Li Internal Alchemy is only one. However, no practice is truly isolated,

---

\*Bracketed text added: The spiritual infant is born when the Internal Alchemical embryo reaches maturity and is ready to form the spiritual body.

†Mantak Chia and Andrew Jan, *The Practice of Greater Kan and Li* (Rochester, Vt.: Destiny Books, 2014), 4–5.

and the practice of Internal Alchemy often includes teachings related to External Alchemy, religious Taoism, ritual, ceremony, magic, shamanism, herbs, dieting, and Chi Kung as well. While isolated pockets of these various traditions occurred simultaneously and in different geographical locations, much overlap and interchange occurs among them. Although any attempt to place the different sects in a linear order is artificial, this format is still useful for the novice reader wishing to gain early insight into the origins of the Universal Healing Tao formulas. Furthermore, the serious adept can draw upon the successes and power of prior masters. Such knowledge of these masters is paramount.

We hope that our effort to situate the UHT practices among the various traditions within Taoism will stimulate readers to embrace the historical aspects of the Taoist inner arts. Novices and advanced practitioners alike can vitalize their meditation practices by further researching and referring to the classics of Taoist thought.

This chapter summarizes the historical movements prior to Bodhidharma's time, which were discussed in greater detail in *The Practice of Greater Kan and Li*. The chapter then goes on to describe pertinent historical developments after the time of Bodhidharma. Note that all the traditions probably have roots in shamanism and the pre-Han era, though those roots may be more or less evident in a given school. While individual schools may have prioritized specific practices, other methods were certainly used in conjunction.

Shamanism: Legendary Shaman Yu (3000 BCE)

Philosophical Taoism: Lao-tzu and Chuang-tzu (600–400 BCE)

Religious Taoism (Purification, Ceremony, and Magic): Zhang Dao-Ling (34–156 CE)

External Alchemy (Taiqing Taoism): Wei Po-Yang (25–220 CE) and Ge Hong (283–343 CE)

Talisman Magic (Sacred Spirit/Ling Bao Taoism):
400–700 CE

Internal Alchemy (Shanqing Taoism): Tao Hong-Jin
(456–536 CE)

Herbal Medicine and Fasting: Tao Hong-Jin revises the Shen
Nong Ben Cao Jing

Sexual Practices (The Arts of the Bedroom Chamber): Su Nu
Ching (~100–400 CE)

Tao Yin and Chi Kung: Bodhidharma (500–600 CE)

Immortals Chong Li-Chuan and Lu Dong-Pin (755 CE)

Complete Reality School (Quanzhen): Wang Chong-Yang
(1113–1170 CE)

Dragon Gate Taoism (Longmen): Qiu Chu-Ji
(1148–1227 CE), Liu I-Ming (1734–1821)

The Universal Healing Tao System: Yi Eng (1867–1967 CE)

The Universal Healing Tao System: Mantak Chia (1944–
present)

# SHAMANISM

## Legendary Shaman Yu
## (3000 BCE)

Shamans like the legendary Yu would enter into altered states of mind through dance or herbs and dialogue with deities, animals, the dream world, the weather, and celestial realms. Even at that time, connection with and journey to the Big Dipper was an important practice. Modern-day Taoist practice appears to have retained many of its shamanic roots.

# PHILOSOPHICAL TAOISM

## Lao-tzu and Chuang-tzu
## (600–400 BCE)

Lao-tzu (604 BCE) is credited as the founder of Taoism and is honored as a deity among the Three Pure Ones. He articulated the essence of Internal Alchemical practice, describing immortality as a consequence of merging the body's multiple spirit and soul entities. He said, "Can you nurture your souls by holding them in unity with the One?"[2] He also reiterated the importance of becoming like a baby in order to achieve the state of mind necessary to comprehend the Tao. He emphasized the sexual nature of enlightenment, describing the "mating of Heaven and Earth" within the meditator's body. In this practice, the adept would act as the female and receive the yang of the heavens. Lao-tzu says, "Opening and closing the gates of heaven, can you play the role of a woman?"[3]

Quotations like these provide enough evidence to demonstrate that the principle of Kan and Li dates back to this early period. Furthermore, we can see that much of Taoist philosophy is based on its mystical roots, rather than on purely intellectual ideas.

Chuang-tzu (369–286 BCE) claimed to be a follower of Lao-tzu. He reputedly refused offers of wealth and fame in order to lead a simple life and articulated the principle of merging the awake and dream worlds. This is seen in his butterfly quote, in which he is unsure, after waking, whether he is a butterfly dreaming he is Chuang-tzu or the other way around. Even in these early times, we find philosophers such as Chuang-tzu documenting successful immortals, including their methods with Pi Gu (a grainless diet).

# RELIGIOUS TAOISM
# (PURIFICATION, CEREMONY, AND MAGIC)

## Zhang Dao-Ling (34–156 CE)

Zhang Dao-Ling brought Taoism to the people. He is credited with enabling access to the goals of longevity through ceremony, ritual, and a code of conduct rather than through the harsh ascetic meditation practices that were accessible to only a chosen few. Now immortality could be achieved by accumulating merit through good deeds, instead of through Inner Alchemy alone. Accumulated merit would eventually rid the follower of the Three Worms and earn him a place in heaven. Zhang's Five Pecks of Rice sect survives today as Zheng Yi Taoism.

# EXTERNAL ALCHEMY
# (TAIQING TAOISM)

## Wei Po-Yang (25–220 CE)
## and Ge Hong (283–343 CE)

Wei Po-Yang was the author of the *Triplex Unity* (Zhouyi Can Tong Qi), likely the oldest book on alchemy. In *The Practice of Greater Kan and Li* we described the legend of Wei Po-Yang and his External Alchemical elixir: although the potion killed his dog, Wei nevertheless proceeded to ingest it and became immortal.

The *Triplex Unity* has its roots in the I Ching. It is here that some of the concepts of Kan and Li were developed. Heaven is replaced with Li, which corresponds to mercury, and Earth is replaced with Kan, which corresponds to lead. The aim of External Alchemy is to find True Lead and True Mercury. This is akin to extracting Heaven out of Kan and Earth out of Li. When True Lead and True Mercury combine then the Golden Elixir can be made.

Ge Hong had prowess as an alchemist and a practitioner, and he was able to achieve immortal status. Internal Alchemists—ourselves included—are indebted to this man not only for his practice but also for his scholarly dedication to the investigation and documentation of alchemy and associated practices. He wrote the *The Master Who Embraces Simplicity* (Bao Pu Tzu) and the *Biographies of Spirit Immortals* (Shen Xian Zhuan). It is these works that give us both insight and the practical methods used by successful immortals from ancient times.

Taiqing Taoism had two basic formulas, which are summarized in the tables below. One formula relied on five-element correspondences and the other on the yin/yang dynamic of mercury and lead.

## THE FIVE-ELEMENT APPROACH TO THE EXTERNAL ALCHEMICAL ELIXIR

| ELEMENT | CHEMICAL | COLOR |
|---------|----------|-------|
| Earth | Realgar or orpiment (arsenic sulphide) | Yellow |
| Fire | Cinnabar (mercuric oxide) | Red |
| Metal | Arsenolite (arsenic oxide) or alum (aluminium oxide) | White |
| Wood | Malachite (copper carbonate) | Green/blue |
| Water | Magnetite (iron oxide) | Black |

## THE YIN/YANG (KAN-AND-LI) APPROACH TO THE ALCHEMICAL ELIXIR

| COMPONENT | PLANETARY INFLUENCE[4] | MYTHICAL INFLUENCE | EXTRACTED |
|-----------|------------------------|--------------------|-----------|
| Red cinnabar (mercuric sulphide) | Sun essence | Dragon | Mercury (grease of dragons) |
| Black lead (native lead) | Moon essence | Tiger | Silver (essence of tiger) |

# TALISMAN MAGIC
# (SACRED SPIRIT/LING BAO TAOISM)

## (400–700 CE)

Sacred Spirit (Ling Bao) Taoism was an intermediate movement that included shamanic and religious elements. It included talisman magic, invocation of deities, and mapping of the occult realm. It blended Buddhist structure with Taoist deities. Sacred Spirit Taoism is marked by the text *The Five Talismans* (Wu Fu Jing) by Ge Chao-Fu. Ge belonged to Ge Hong's family lineage and was his grand-nephew. This text emphasized many aspects of Chi Kung, as well as methods of achieving immortality via the ingesting of chi rather than with External Alchemical techniques. The formula for Invocation of the Three Pure Ones described in chapter 4 is likely to have been developed in this movement. Ling Bao Taoism gradually diminished in popularity, but many of its practices were absorbed into Shanqing Taoism.

# INTERNAL ALCHEMY
# (SHANQING TAOISM)

## Tao Hong-Jin (456–536 CE)

In Shanqing (Highest Clarity) Taoism we find the first solid roots of the UHT system. While remnants of the preceding movements are still traceable, there is a huge thrust at this time toward Inner Alchemy. Notably, we see in this movement the solidification of the concepts of inner deities and spirits;[5] the unification of these inner souls and spirits is central to forming the spiritual body. Furthermore, it was Shanqing Taoism that perfected spirit flight, which requires the formation of a spiritual body. With this flight comes connection to and absorption of planetary and stellar bodies. We find in this Higher Clarity movement very detailed formulas on how these practices are achieved. Some meditations, like the

Microcosmic Orbit and Guarding the One (see more on Guarding the One at the end of this chapter), have similarities to our current practice. Likewise many of the Chi Kung exercises such as Elixir Chi Kung also have their roots in this movement. Many of the practices of Shanqing Taoism were adopted by the Complete Reality school (Quanzhen),[6] which is closely related to the Universal Healing Tao system.

## HERBAL MEDICINE AND FASTING

### Tao Hong-Jin (456–536 CE)

Tao Hong-Jin revised the Materia Medica. His work documents the medicinal and spiritual properties of over seven hundred herbs. Herbs were important for immortal practice as they could improve an adept's health and subsequently support the harsher demands of a Pi Gu diet and fasting.

Some of the Chinese herbs used by successful immortals include: Shu (Atractylis), Tianmen Dong (Asparagus Root), Shang Lu (Poke Root), Pine derivatives, Ling Zhi (Reishi Mushrooms), Gan Cao (Licorice Root), Chang Pu (Sweet flag/Calamus), Huang Jing (Solomon's Seal). Pi Gu is best translated as the "absence of grains," although some interpret it as complete fasting. Practitioners who emphasized diet include Li Chun-Yun (1677 [or 1736]–1933), who allegedly lived over two hundred years and had twenty-three wives.[7]

## THE ARTS OF THE BEDROOM CHAMBER (FAN ZHONG)

### Su Nu Ching (~100–400 CE)

In most traditions, sexual practices alone were considered a valid path toward immortality. *The Immaculate Girl* says, "If you can avoid mortification and injury and attain the arts of sex, you will have found the way of non-death."[8] Peng Zu (1900–1066 BCE) is the most renowned advocate of the sexual arts who achieved immortal status as an earth-bound transcendent. His methods included a combination of semen retention, Chi Kung, and absorption of vital yin essence from his partners. He was a critic of the austere practices of celibate monks.[9]

However, the sexual path had its darker aspects, with some practitioners practicing a sexual form of vampirism rather than seeking dual enlightenment.

Sexuality and Kan and Li practice are so interconnected that it is hard to separate them. The training and events in the bedroom (including self-stimulation) provide the framework upon which the more ascetic tradition can be based. The experiences of orgasm form the core techniques for Kan and Li practice, and the vocabulary for Kan and Li is based on many aspects of sexuality itself. Practices like "self-intercourse," the "merging of yin and yang," "giving birth," and "insemination of the spirit" can be better understood after sexual practice in the physical world.

The Inner Alchemical world derives its meaning from the actuality of sexuality and reproductive life on this planet. The only difference is that it is experienced and summarized in energetic form within the body and mind of the practitioner.

## TAO YIN AND CHI KUNG

### Bodhidharma (500–600 CE)

Separating Tao Yin and Chi Kung from any tradition, including Kan and Li practice, is problematic. Most sects practiced some physical exercise that involved the use of chi. Notables who advocated physical Chi Kung or Tao Yin activities included Hua To (140–208 CE) and Bodhidharma (500–600 CE). Hua To created the *Five Animal Tao Yin* (Wu Qin Xi), while Bodhidharma wrote the *Muscle Changing Classic* (Yi Jin Jing) and the *Bone Marrow Washing Classic* (Xi Sui Jin).

## IMMORTALS CHONG LI-CHUAN
## AND LU DONG-PIN

Lu Dong-Pin and Chong Li-Chuan are inseparable from Taoist doctrine and ritual. Their works are fundamental to philosophy and practice.

## Chong Li-Chuan

Chong Li-Chuan (fig. 1.1) lived during the Han dynasty. He is one of the celebrated Eight Immortals and a patriach of the Quanzhen sect (see page 14). Chong was a respected general in the Han army, but following a humiliating defeat, he decided to search for new meaning in his life. Later, he met a sage in the Zhong Nan Mountains who would turn his life around.

Chong's new life was devoted to the spiritual development of others rather than to the death and destruction of soldiers and communities. He was portrayed in his later years much like the Buddha with a large bare belly, a bald head, and a beard. He is credited with coauthorship of *The Teachings of the Tao as Transmitted by Chung and Lu* (Chung Lu Chuan Tao Chi).* He achieved immortality, transcended time, and gave instructions in dream form to Lu Dong-Pin five hundred years later.

## Lu Dong-Pin (755 CE)

Lu Dong-Pin (fig. 1.2) was a member of the Tang Emperor's family. His initial name was Li, but he changed it to Lu to avoid identification with the overthrown emperor. He did not want to risk being murdered by associates of the new female emperor, Wu Ze-Tian.

After Lu met Chong Li-Chuan in a vision, he subsequently had a dream of alternate futures. One involved a high-ranking position that held acclaim. In this future he married a beautiful woman and had two

---

*As was the tradition in many Taoist schools, teachings that were transmitted via dreams or meditation were attributed to the apparition, so Chong Li-Chuan is considered a coauthor of these texts.

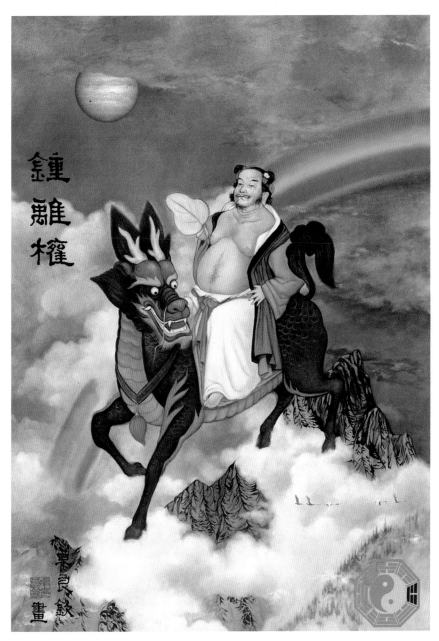

鍾離權

Fig. 1.1. Chong Li-Chuan

children, but his status created envy and his family was slaughtered. Lu thus decided not to pursue status or a beautiful partner. Instead, he chose to become a student of Chong Li-Chuan and devote himself to Inner

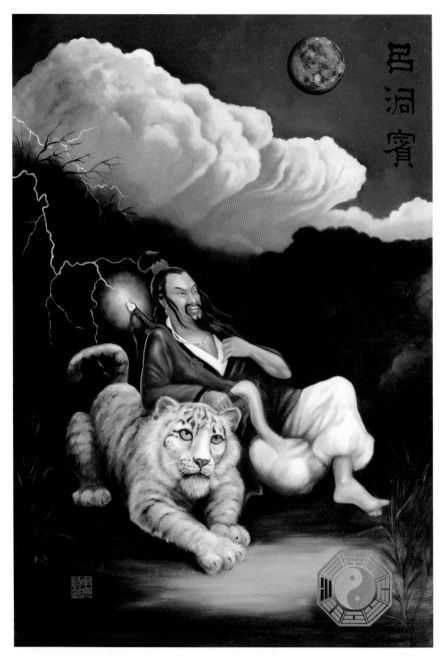

Fig. 1.2. Lu Dong-Pin

Alchemy. Lu learned alchemical and sexual teachings from Chong Li-Chuan in 815 CE.

Lu Dong-Pin is credited with authorship of multiple texts, including *The Secrets of the Golden Flower, The Teachings of the Tao as Transmitted by Chung and Lu, The True Manual of Perfected Equalization* (Chi Chi Chen Ching), and *The Taoist Patriarch Lu Dong-Pin's Five Poetical Essays on Sexual Technique* (Lu Tsu Wu Phien). Lu Dong-Pin achieved the status of Celestial Immortal and also lived on the earth for over four hundred years. Like his teacher, he is one of the eight Taoist immortals and a patriarch of the Quanzhen sect.

## Chong and Lu in Taoist Doctrine

As immortals, both Chong Li-Chuan and Lu Dong-Pin are associated with particular aspects of Taoist doctrine. Some of their correspondences are shown in the table below.

### CHARACTERISTICS OF THE IMMORTALS CHONG AND LU

|  | CHONG LI-CHUAN | LU DONG-PIN |
|---|---|---|
| **Trigram** | Zheng (thunder) | Tui (lake) |
| **Emblem** | Fan that resurrects the dead | Sword (for conquering ignorance and temptations), horsehair whisk (ability to fly on clouds) |
| **Birthday** | Fifteenth day of the fourth month | April 14 |
| **Animal** | Chimera (hybrid flying animal), white crane (symbolizing immortality) | White Tiger from Goddess of West |
| **Body** | Bald head, large abdomen | Three-part beard signifies the three Thrusting Channels |

# COMPLETE REALITY SCHOOL (QUANZHEN)

## Wang Chong-Yang (1113–1170 CE)

Quanzhen Taoism can be translated as "The Way of Completeness and Truth." It is also known as the Complete Reality school. The focus of this school was on Internal Alchemy. It prioritized an ascetic life with focus on solitary reclusive practice. The goals of the school were for its adepts to achieve health, longevity, and immortality.

The founder of the school was Wang Chong-Yang (1113–1170 CE) (fig. 1.3). He practiced alone for seven years in the Zhong Nan Mountains, which had been housing Taoist hermits since the Qin dynasty. In the mountains, Wang met apparitions of Lu Dong-Pin and Chong Li-Chuan in 1159 and 1160. They trained him in the secret arts of Internal Alchemy and provided him with instructions as to his future teachings.

Wang consequently dedicated his school to these immortals (along with Liu Hai-Chan). Some allege that it was he who wrote *The Secrets of the Golden Flower*. However, as mentioned earlier, students would attribute texts to the teacher if they had come via spiritual transmission. Wang had seven disciples, of which Qiu Chi-Ji is the most notable as he started the Dragon Gate (Longmen) sect.

Quanzhen appeared as a monastic order around 1170 CE.[10] Since then, the Quanzhen school has held variable status. There were times when it was in disfavor with the ruling government of the time and had to be overtly abandoned. Consequently, teachings were sometimes held in lay venues. At other times, Quanzhen masters took over ruined Buddhist temples and even held leadership positions in the Confucian schools. Just prior to the Yuan dynasty (1271–1368), Taoist scholars compiled the Taoist canon, to which the Quanzhen school contributed approximately sixty works.

Quanzhen is generally regarded as the official form of Taoism. Its

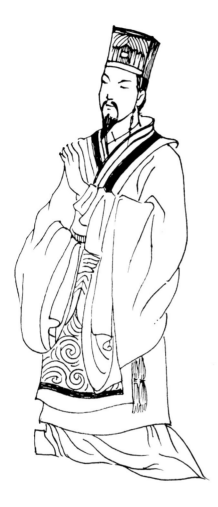

Fig. 1.3. Wang Chong-
Yang, founder of the
Quanzhen sect

predominant focus was Nei Dan (Internal Alchemy), within the setting
of a monastic or an isolated existence. Its practitioners included many
women (up to a third). During the Yuan dynasty there were approximately four thousand monasteries; today the Taoist society claims
twenty thousand adepts. The Bai Yun Guan (White Cloud Temple)
is a well-known temple in Beijing that is still active with Quanzhen
teachings.

Quanzhen had a Northern school (*bei zong*) and a Southern school
(*nan zong*). The founder of the Southern school was Chan Po-Tuan

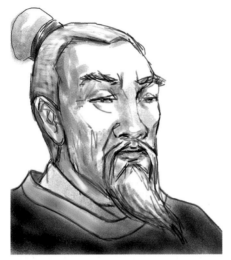

Fig. 1.4. Chang Po-Tuan, founder of the Quanzhen Southern school.

(987–1082 CE) (fig. 1.4), who wrote *Awakening to Reality* (Wu Zhen Pian). The Southern school is less ascetic than the Northern school and retained the sexual teachings as taught by Lu Dong-Pin.

## DRAGON GATE TAOISM (LONGMEN)

### Qiu Chu-Ji (1148–1227 CE)

The Longmen tradition was founded by Qiu Chu-Ji, a disciple of Wang Chong-Yang. This school was an offshoot of the northern branch of the Quanzhen school. It further developed Taoist Inner Alchemy by blending it with teachings from Buddhist and Confucian schools. Of course, this fusion of religious traditions had been occurring since the foundation of the Quanzhen school. The blend of Taoism and Buddhism is particularly noted in the Quanzhen text *The Secrets of the Golden Flower.* Together with Spirit writing the teachings from Lu Dong-Pin it is claimed that this led to the classic written by Longmen adepts in 1668.[11]

The survival of the school was ensured in the troubled times of the thirteenth century when Qiu Chu-Ji negotiated a protective order from Genghis Khan in 1222 CE.[12]

From the end of the Ming dynasty (1368–1644), adepts of the Quanzhen school often prided themselves on belonging to the Longmen tradition.[13] Under the direction of Wang Kun-Yang (?–1680), Longmen scholars organized monasteries and developed a genuine school.[14] On the surface, the teachings appeared to imply that Inner Alchemy was an inferior path open to adepts who sought longevity and immortality for vain reasons alone.[15] However, Wang Kun-Yang and others firmly believed that the enlightened mind, strengthened by Inner Alchemy training, could change and heal the world. Wang Kun-Yang reemphasized the importance of healing communities and nations in line with Buddhist and Confucian ideals.

The Longmen tradition allowed local communities to keep their unique traditions.[16] The monks of Chang Bai-Shan—including Yi Eng and his master—were part of the Longmen school, but they retained some of their local teachings, formulas, and traditions.

## Liu I-Ming (1734–1821)

Liu I-Ming was an eleventh-generation Taoist master of the Dragon Gate sect (fig. 1.5). He began his life in poor health but turned it around using Taoist methods. He studied Taoist alchemy, the I Ching, Chinese medicine, Confucianism, and Buddhism, and made immense contributions to written literature. The main Kan and Li texts contain multiple references to Liu's works and commentaries. Without his writings our understanding of alchemy would be significantly lessened.

Liu I-Ming's contributions include:

- His own version of the I Ching from an alchemical (Kan and Li) perspective. He was a recognized master of the I Ching.

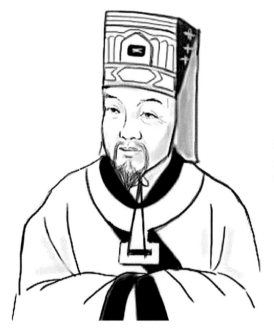

Fig. 1.5. Liu I-Ming, master of the Dragon Gate sect

- *Preface to the Pointers* (Zhin An Zhen Xu). Liu I-Ming was a true mystic who saw all religions as one. This text was about finding commonality within the three major Chinese religions of Taoism, Buddhism, and Confucianism.
- *Nine Essentials for the Cultivation of Perfection* (Xiu Zhen Jiu Yao). A text about seeking perfection through the Tao.
- *Book of Passing through Barriers* (Tong Guan Wen). This text included advice for overcoming barriers such as sexual desire in achieving spiritual development.

Liu also wrote insightful and useful commentaries on many key texts, including the following:

- *Awakening to Reality* (Wu Zhian Pian) by Chang Po-Tuan.
- *Inner Teachings of Taoism* (Jin Dan Si Bai Zi), by Chang Po-Tuan.
- *Triplex Unity* (Zhouyi Can Tong Qi) by Wei Po-Yang.

- *Yellow Emperor's Book of Secret Correspondences* (Yin Fu Jing), author unknown.

Many of these works would likely have remained opaque to understanding without Liu I-Ming's contribution.

## Principles of the Dragon Gate School

The Dragon Gate school emphasized the fluidity of practice, teaching that once the formulas for the Microcosmic Orbit and Kan and Li practice had been learned, the practitioner should let the formulas go. In this view, the process of setting up detailed anatomical energetic blueprints within the formulas is only a transitory exercise. To this point, Taoism scholar Monica Esposito says, "In the practice of the Microcosmic Orbit or Path of Men, the adept works on places in the body that play the role of physical markers. These physical markers are like "fingers pointing at the moon" and are used for supporting the practice at the outset. Once their function has been fulfilled, they must be abandoned."[17]

The Longmen tradition taught that immortality—including finding the Macrocosmic Orbit—was a result of nonaction. Practitioners believed that it is in the space between the intercourse of Kan and Li that the mystery converts all of time and space into one experience.[18]

The Dragon Gate branch of Quanzhen is thriving today. Well-known masters include Wang Li Ping (1949–present). He teaches techniques from *The Secrets of the Golden Flower* and *The Complete Methods of Numinous Treasure* (Lingbao Bifa), another text attributed to Chong Li-Chuan and Lu Dong-Pin's system of Internal Alchemy.[19]

# THE UNIVERSAL HEALING TAO SYSTEM

## Yi Eng (1867–1967 CE)

Before Yi Eng (fig. 1.6) met his final and most capable teacher he had already spent thirty years studying Inner Alchemy with various masters from different sects. An abbot of a northern Dragon Gate temple then advised Yi Eng to further his Inner Alchemical practice and learn the genuine immortal Nei Dan practices.[20] To achieve this, he was to leave and seek a competent master in the mountains of Chang Bai Shan (Ever White Mountains).

The Chang Bai Shan are located in the Jilin and Liaoning provinces between China and North Korea. The mountains here had the reputation of fostering high-level immortal practitioners because of the unique blend of Ching, chi, and shen found in the herbs growing there. There is little specifically written about the hermits that practiced in this area, but we know that the Longmen tradition both tolerated and

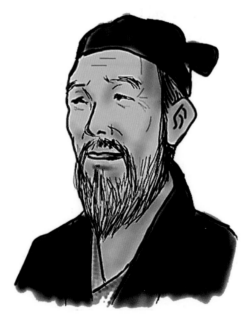

Fig. 1.6. Master Yi Eng,
Mantak Chia's teacher

dialogued with traditions in their local vicinity. It is likely that there was overlap or shared practices between the monastic residents of local temples and the hermits of Chang Bai Shan.

In a cave within these mountains, Yi Eng found the master who had allegedly forgotten his name. The master was in a deep out-of-body meditation with his body in suspended animation. Yi Eng realized that his first task was to protect the master from insects and animals while he was in this state. On occasion, the master returned to his body and began teaching Yi Eng. Over three years, Yi Eng learned the formulas that are currently taught today in the Universal Healing Tao (UHT) system, including:

1. The Inner Smile, Six Healing Sounds, the Microcosmic Orbit, and Chi Kung
2. Sexual Practices including Dual Cultivation
3. The Fusion practices and the Macrocosmic Orbit
4. Lesser Enlightenment of the Kan and Li
5. Greater Enlightenment of the Kan and Li
6. Greatest Enlightenment of the Kan and Li
7. Sealing of the Five Senses
8. Congress of Heaven and Earth
9. Reunion of Heaven and Man

Perhaps as a consequence of the Cultural Revolution, Yi Eng traveled down from the North through to the South, where he resided in the mountains outside of Hong Kong. He was ninety-one in 1958, when he first met Mantak Chia, who was then fourteen years old. Yi Eng taught the nine formulas to this young yet devoted and capable adept. He instructed Mantak Chia to learn human anatomy and to teach these formulas to the West. Yi Eng died in Bangkok nine years later, at the age of one hundred (1967).

## CONTEXTUALIZING YI ENG'S PRACTICES

Historians such as Miller regard Yi Eng as a hermit practitioner of the Dragon Gate division of the Quanzhen Northern school.[21] However, the actual formulas taught to Yi Eng by a hermit in the Ever White Mountains are variant from the orthodox practices of the Dragon Gate sect.

In the bigger picture, all the practices can be classified as belonging to the Chong-Lu tradition. These in turn relate to practices developed in the Shanqing schools and prior. Over the years the formulas have remained steadfast, although interpretations and ultimate endpoints are fluid. Interpretation has changed with Master Chia's deeper understanding of the practices over the years. Furthermore, with increasing numbers of Taoist texts translated into English and the knowledge base of esoteric Inner Alchemy ever expanding, a dialogue ensues which enables an evolution of understanding.

Yi Eng's formulas have many themes and practices that are similar to Inner Alchemical formulas in other Taoist traditions. While UHT practitioners should always attempt to preserve Yi Eng's formulas, the principle of comparing and contrasting them to other practices is a valuable one. Such comparisons provide a freshness that helps to revitalize practices that have been repeated verbatim for prolonged periods of time. It also promotes an opportunity for like-minded adepts from different Inner Alchemy traditions to learn from each other and propagate the healing aspects of this profound discipline.

In the following sections we will compare a few of Yi Eng's formulas to the larger context of the Taoist Inner Alchemy tradition. Specifically we will look at Sitting in Forgetfulness, Guarding the One, and the Whirlwind. Comparisons of Kan and Li will be made repeatedly through the book.

## The Inner Smile

The Inner Smile is a cornerstone practice of Yi Eng's nine formulas. It overlaps with other mystical practices including Christian mystical practice and Buddhism, as well as with practices from other Taoist traditions

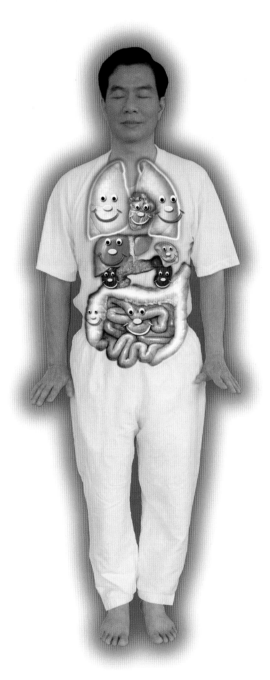

Fig. 1.7. The Inner Smile has elements of
Sitting in Forgetfulness and Guarding the One.

(fig. 1.7). The Inner Smile is used as a starting point for all higher practices. It is a simple method of dissolving and merging disparate energies (polar energies) into one experience of Primordial Chi.

The Inner Smile practice reiterates the foundation principle of the Taoist creation story: the primordial gave rise to yin and yang and then to the Three Pure Ones, the five elements, and the ten thousand things. Capturing this Primordial Chi and letting all energies, experiences, and phenomena dissolve and return into it is the fundamental goal of practice. As all energies both pleasant and unpleasant merge with the primordial, the body dissolves and merges with everything. Michael Winn compares this to the eighth-century Taoist practice of Sitting in Forgetfulness (Zuowang).[22]

### *Zuowang (Sitting in Forgetfulness):* 混合

Zuowang is a Quanzhen practice. Its principle is one of undoing and returning to the primordial (or the Wu Wei) without effort. Zuowang can be interpreted as letting go to the diversified energies and ultimately into the bliss of the primordial. There is no doing, as the sitter forgets by turning off intellectual thought and entering the moment of sensual awareness. His or her former and future existence dissolve into the diversified energies, which eventually coalesce as a singular experience. Zuowang ends up with a positive embrace of the primordial space of the Wu Wei without effort.[23] It can be equated to the Christian principle of forgiveness and acceptance: all energies are welcome to return to God, just as all energies return to the Primordial Chi. Because this sitting while letting go is so blissful and rejuvenating, the adept will have no alternative but to smile.

### *Shouyi (Guarding the One):* 守一

Shouyi is another interpretation of the Inner Smile practice. Like the Inner Smile, Guarding the One is regarded as a foundation for all higher-level meditation practice. At the same time, it is sufficient on its own for achieving immortality.[24] Guarding the One can be traced back to Ge Hong's time and is documented in the *Bao Pu Zu*.

In Ge Hong's time, Shouyi included a systematic formula that visualized the pleasant "inner light of the One" passing from the head to the specific organs such as the heart, lungs, and kidneys.[25] There is also mention of merging the tripartite division of awareness into one. This correlates with the latter sequence of the Inner Smile that merges the three minds into one mind and with the merging of the three tan tiens, including the notions of spirit, chi and Ching. Ge Hong also cites merging the three main senses of sight, hearing, and the subtle (smell or the breath).[26]

The *Scripture of the Great Peace* (Taiping Jing), which also dates from the Han era, highlights the principle of concentration by focusing the mind on the pleasant yin or primordial sensation of chi and not letting that go! The scripture says, "In a state of complete concentration, when the light first arises, make sure you hold on to it and never let go."[27] During the Tang dynasty, this practice reverted more to Zuowang with its apophatic principle of undoing and forgetting that which is conditioned. The practice becomes one of recovering that which is already in us.[28] In Shanqing Taoism during the Sui and Tang eras, the Shouyi "appears to be mainly a fight against strong [negative] emotions."[29] This principle echoes the Inner Smile's cultivation of courage, love, kindness, openness, and gentleness.

## Fusion (Hun He) or Whirlwind (Hui Feng)

The roots of Fusion practice date all the way back to Shanqing Taoism (fig. 1.8). Isabelle Robinet explains Fusion or Hun He as a return of multiplicity to the One.[30] The *Scripture of the Great Purity* (Shangqing Ching), the central scripture of Shangqing Taoism, refers to Fusion practice wherein the three tan tiens become one and the five sectors of all phenomena are fused. Chinese terms such as *hun tung* or *hun hui* were used to signify fusion of the hundred spirits.[31] Like the UHT Fusion of the Five Elements, the Hun He practice includes a reversal of the Taoist creation theory. The reversal is called the "whirlwind" (*hui feng*). "[The] whirlwind is at the beginning of the body's return to life" and "liberates

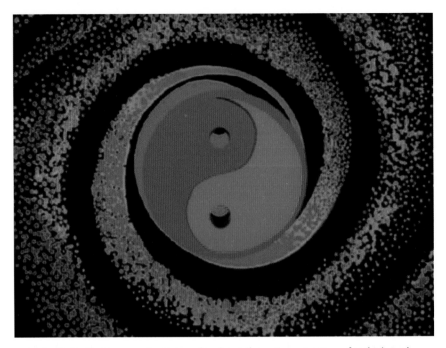

Fig. 1.8. Fusion practice traces back to Shanqing practice of Whirlwind.

(one) from death."[32] Other researchers interpret Fusion as a whirlpool of internal energies.[33] The turning of the Tai Chi symbol in the UHT practice is like a whirlwind that returns the adept to the beginning and results in fetal consciousness and rebirth.

The concepts of Fusion are alluded to in Lu Dong-Pin's writings, when he discusses returning to the elixir through a merging of the five elements and all their correspondences in the body.[34] The Dragon Gate sect relied similarly on the five elements, connecting them on the earthly plane and in the solar system as a method of training. This practice is called the Jewel Powers practice and the Three Immortalist Exercise practices.[35]

## Kan and Li

Much of the remainder of this book is dedicated to exploring the development of Kan and Li practice in the original classics. See the appendix on pages 227–29 for a detailed listing of the relevant texts.

The Universal Healing Tao system has a strong connection to the Chong Lu tradition; remember that the Quanzhen sect acknowledges Lu Dong-Pin and Chong Li-Chuan as their patriarchs. Therefore practices must continually attempt to realign with their teachings both via the written word in the classics and via other methods such as channelling spiritual writings. Furthermore, recall that Yi Eng could be classified as a hermit of the Dragon Gate branch of the Quanzhen school.[36]

The most relevant text for Kan and Li practice is Lu Dong-Pin's *The Teachings of the Tao as Transmitted by Chung and Lu* (Chong Lu Chuan Tao Chi). It is similar in principle to the *Triplex Unity* and the *Dragon Tiger Classic* of the Han era.[37] In this text of Chung and Lu, the meditation of Kan and Li is regarded as a vehicle for achieving immortality.[38] Descriptions of the meditation in this classic include applying the fire and the water, self-intercourse, the dragon occupying the house of Li and the tiger occupying the house of Kan, steaming (vapor), production of essence (condensation of steam), the Waterwheel, and collection of sun and moon energy.

In modern Dragon Gate practice, Wang Li-Ping's students say:

> Those who are highly cultivated use the pure energies of the external five elements to nurture pure energy (Primordial Chi) inside the body, opposing the operation of nature to rise above it, combining fire and water, producing and culling medicine, crystalizing the alchemical elixir and incubating it, thus becoming immortals.[39]

There is no doubt that the UHT practices of Kan and Li have roots and connections to the aforementioned classics and other Quanzhen sects. It is our hope that serious students will read these classics and reflect on their similarities and differences in order to gain insight and develop their personal practice.

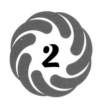

# Why Practice the Greatest Kan and Li Meditation?

*When true yin and true yang are blended, the mechanism of life therein wells forth and congeals into a spiritual embryo, coming into being from nonbeing, from being into nonbeing escaping the illusory body, and bringing forth the real body: only then can one share the eternity of heaven and earth.*

LIU I-MING[1]

There are several reasons for practicing the Kan and Li meditations. Some of the potential benefits of practice were addressed in *The Practice of Greater Kan and Li*—namely health, long life, and freedom. These aims are summarized below, though the reader is advised to read the full text for more information.* In addition to the benefits already mentioned, two further goals of practicing the Greatest Kan and Li formulae in particular are: discovering the truth and achieving immortality.

---

*Mantak Chia and Andrew Jan, *The Practice of Greater Kan and Li* (Rochester, Vt.: Destiny Books, 2014).

# HEALTH

Most of the health benefits of Kan and Li practice are a result of opening the lower tan tien. Almost all channels flow when the lower tan tien is opened, including the Microcosmic Orbit (Governing and Functional Channels), the Belt Channels, the Thrusting Channels, and—with the assistance of the Lesser Kan and Li practice—also the Bridge and Regulator channels. Maximum channel flow leads to optimum function and ideal exchange with Air Chi, Food Chi, Heaven and Earth Chi, True Chi, Wei Chi, and Ying Chi. In this way the body realizes its ideal functioning and homeostasis.

Unfortunately, there is no good evidence from Western medicine to support meditation as a therapeutic modality. This lack of good clinical data may discourage some aspiring adepts. It should be noted, however, that the existing studies are focused mainly on patients with anxiety or neurotic disorders, rather than on the loftier goals of our readership.

There is some clinical support for the idea that Tai Chi and Chi Kung can have a positive influence on health. The fact that some of these studies achieved positive results even with randomized and short-course trials is reassuring. Ultimately, however, it is hard to "prove" anything about an Inner Alchemy practice that has been a tradition for thousands of years.

## The Eight Pillars of Health

The Eight Pillars of health are Chi Kung and Meditation, Good Sleep and Rest, Good Food and Digestion, Good Water, Balanced Emotions, Loving Sexuality/Relationship, Good Vocation, and Good Spiritual Connections (fig. 2.1). These pillars have been discussed in some detail in several previous UHT titles, including *The Practice of Greater Kan and Li* and *Tai Chi Wu Style*.

Kan and Li practice can have positive affects on all of these pillars, as is summarized below.

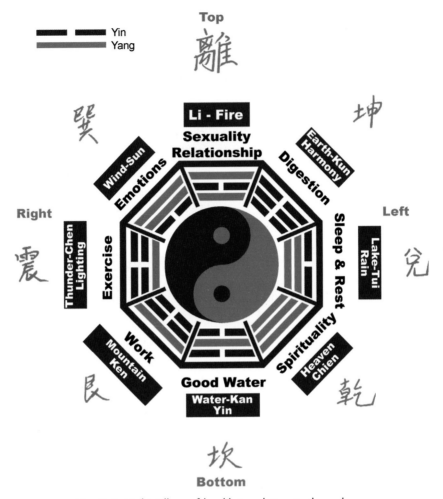

Fig. 2.1. Eight Pillars of health in relation to the pakua

### Chi Kung and Meditation

Because Kan and Li is a form of Chi Kung and is a high-level meditation, improvements in these practices are a given. Figure 2.2 shows how Kan and Li practice promotes health according to the principles of traditional Chinese medicine. By increasing the amount of Heavenly and Earth Chi and expanding the lower tan tien, the adept's health is likely to improve.

### Good Sleep and Rest

In *The Practice of Greater Kan and Li* we discussed the three worlds of mortal life: the meditation world, the dream world, and the everyday

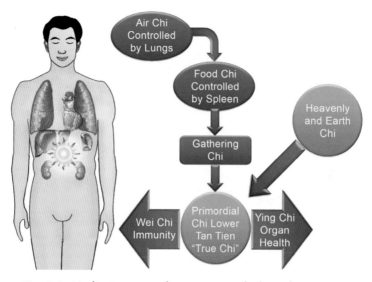

Fig. 2.2. Meditation can enhance Postnatal Chi in the tan tien.

world. Kan and Li practice helps bring the meditation world to everyday consciousness, which has many important benefits for sleep and rest.

Firstly, Kan and Li practice helps us atttune to the innermost aspects of our being. These aspects can be described as energies, souls, and spirits. One realizes that harmonizing the internal milieu has little to do with fame, wealth, or entertainment. The lessons learned in harmonizing the internal milieu are gradually applied to the material world. This gradually reduces struggle and conflict within. Without this struggle within there is more space for rest and good sleep. The dream world no longer tries to resolve the unresolvable. Our society and temporal conditioning often wants us to be fragmented. What we think society wants is ultimately impossible.

The dream world provides us with clues about our inner souls and spirits and what we actually want out of this lifetime. The sooner we address these deep inner needs the sooner we can rest. With practice, there is harmony between the three worlds. Dreams become a portal for meditation practice and what to do in the material world. Meditation provides a still point around which all activity revolves. Rest is stillness and without rest we become sick.

## Good Food and Digestion, and Good Water

The process of refinement that occurs in achieving the goals of Kan and Li practice spills over into your worldly life. The modifications to food and digestion that follow from Kan and Li practice are discussed in detail in chapter 7 of this book. Good water is also a must—this you can understand from either an orthodox or an alternative viewpoint. From an orthodox point of view, water can contain pollutants ranging from hazardous chemicals to traces of hormones from livestock supplementation. Alternative understanding is best described by the author Masaru Emoto, who showed how the actual crystalline structure of water is badly affected by negative emotions. Its structure is also denatured when sourced from large industrial cities.[2] Most practitioners find that maintaining a pure internal milieu eventually creates a natural aversion to external pollutants and additives in both food and water.

## Sexual Relations

Kan and Li practice demands that adepts orient their sexual energy to loftier goals rather than primitive ones. These goals include raising the body's personality and frequency to equal those of the benevolent immortals. For men, this intention leads to reduced semen loss and the subsequent retention of Prenatal Chi. Health is consequently maintained and is likely to improve. For women, a consequence of the practice is lighter periods. Without this energy drain, healing can occur and health can move forward.

## Spirituality

Spirituality is a given in Kan and Li practice. By opening the energetic realm within the body and mind, connection to the spiritual realm becomes possible. Furthermore, tools and formulas are provided to enhance harmony within this dimension.

# LONGEVITY

Previously, we discussed longevity as a continuation of good health. If one followed the principles of the Eight Pillars and practiced Kan and Li, one's life span would be expected to extend. However, a doctrine of longevity beyond and inclusive of alchemical practice emerged in the Tang dynasty. This doctrine described a deity called the Director of Allotted Life Spans, who determined the length of each person's life.

The Director determined a person's years by the balance and interplay of two opposing forces—the Three Worms and the Three Pure Ones. The Three Worms advocate for the death wish, while the Three Pure Ones request eternal life. Like yin and yang, these two opposite forces battle and interplay throughout one's life. The aim of the worms is to fragment the person, cultivating chaos and struggle among the different spirits and energies within. The worms manifest their mischief by attacking each of the tan tiens. The infection of the lower tan tien—Peng Jiaou—results in wayward sexuality with loss of semen and menses. Peng Zhi perverts the heart tan tien and encourages it to seek gratification through status, material wealth, and the senses. The upper tan tien is imbalanced by Peng Ju, which incorrectly prioritizes the intellect, scientific and worldly knowledge, and appeasement through the external senses.

The Three Pure Ones—the Jade Emperor, the Cinnabar Sovereign, and the Sovereign King—aim to reverse this fragmentation and orient each person in the direction of the Tao. Sexuality becomes the catalyst and method of reuniting disparate energies. The emotions and organ energy of the lower tan tien can be oriented toward self-sacrifice and unity. In the middle tan tien, the heart begins to regain its original passion of being at one with everything. The upper tan tien uses intellect to support the path, aid observation, and open mystical vision. All three tan tiens wish also to sacrifice their own positions and merge into one as the immortal fetus and infant.

In this way, expelling the Three Worms requires a major reorientation of every facet of existence. It is in large part a matter of choice and self-belief.

# FREEDOM

In *The Practice of Greater Kan and Li* we discussed freedom as the opportunity to acknowledge and release the most disparate sides of ourselves— our earthly and heavenly natures. Our earthly nature includes all our sexual and bestial desires as well as our emotional and material existence. Our heavenly aspects include our virtue, good will, and connectedness, as well as our souls and spirits and all things immaterial.

Freedom also includes the deep desire to be free of the bodily tension that is often created by our work, sleep habits, eating habits, and social interactions. Once we have balanced and merged our opposite polarities and experienced the sensation of an open body, there is no turning back. This state of openness, which many of us crave, is achievable only when we find the right formula for freedom of all aspects of self.

The Kan and Li formulas provide a vehicle for removing habitual tensions and educating all aspects of the self to harmonize. This state of being takes many years of practice and cultivation. Even in the middle of a meditation, tension in the body provides ongoing solid feedback that work needs to be done. In Kan and Li practice, the goals of forming the embryo, completing gestation, and raising a spiritual body require almost all tension to be released.

A new existence is thus called for! It is where the body is full of energy and lacking tension and blockages. Both of these states bring eternal delight. They are pleasing and are a hallmark of the Way.

## Returning to Freedom

Breaking down the shackles of our conditioned mind requires some effort. We need to retrace our steps not only to infancy but back through our fetal origins and beyond. With Kan and Li practice we return to being a newborn babe. We feel our primordial energy and learn to suckle once more. Beyond that we return to the womb and lose our external breath. We re-create the orgasm that conceived us. Finally, we remember our spirit—much like a shooting star—traveling through time and space to incarnate our material existence. Before that, we were truly at peace, whether in our original birth star or the darkness of outer space.

The fall began with our first interaction with the material world. Each successive stage was a further tearing from Heaven down to Earth. However, through the Tao we can find freedom and rise again. The paradox is that we don't really need to "learn"; the energetic memory is already there. It's a matter of unlearning-and-returning via the Kan and Li practice. Breaking the shackles is difficult at times, and entails transformation of the mind. What is right and wrong comes into question. However, truth and freedom ultimately reside in your own body knowledge. This is sensed as openness rather than tension. To be open is to be with the Tao and to be closed is displeasing.

## Taming the Mind

Within Inner Alchemy there are the three major components of mind that need to be identified and ultimately merged and transformed. These components are space, time, and the observer. In our usual Kan and Li teachings we only briefly mention the observer, but it is an important aspect of the teachings of the Dragon Gate school. The transformation of the observer is a key component of taming the mind.

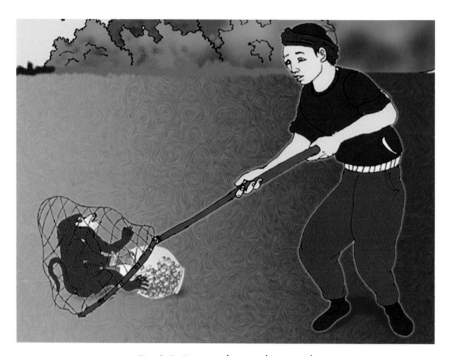

Fig 2.3. Taming the monkey mind

In human affairs our normal arrangement of the human—monkey mind, heart, emotions, and sexuality—involves the following: when the discriminating spirit of the human mind (monkey mind) sees objects and encounters feelings, it flies up. The center that is normally located in the lower tan tien is uprooted, and tension accumulates in the neck and regions of the back. This instability of mind can be a reaction to a variety of things. When the body is sick or contemplating death the mind goes into chaos. It begins a disturbing routine of rumination, obsession, and worry.

The heart can also fall into a state of chaos. It can never know when enough is enough. In its fragmented state separate from the Higher Shen and other spirits within the body, the heart never knows when to stop. It is "like a snake that wants to swallow an elephant":[3] it is avaricious for bathing of the external senses and emotions with entertainment, personal involvement, and accumulation of objects. Upon meeting evil or wrongdoings our emotional body goes into anger and hate mode. We suffer accordingly and even get sick with such reactions.

The desire to escape this reaction is strong. Ultimately we seek to tame the mind and "detach . . . from affairs."[4] We want to appreciate the journey through the human realm but not be attached to it as though it were the only reality. We want to be compassionate but not get caught up with those that suffer. Too many people are "losing their heads" and it is important that someone stands up and leads. This transformation of the observer is what we seek and is obviously another very important reason to do our alchemical practice. The Kan and Li practice provides a very real methodology for accessing this state of mind. For it is through the firing of our human mind (monkey mind) in the cauldron and cooking it that it transforms into the mindless state of the Tao.

# TRUTH

Truth is a classic philosophical goal that, like freedom, has many varied interpretations. From a religious viewpoint, truth involves the dissolving of falsehood such that the ideal can be revealed. In some respects it overlaps with the process of obtaining freedom: the truth is laid bare once temporal conditioning has been removed. For some, the truth is a newly found purpose in a previously chaotic existence. For others, truth is the realization that all the fragments of self can be aligned.

In Taoist thought, Truth is mostly equivalent to the Way. Liu I-Ming says, "When the firing process conforms to what is appropriate, the real solidifies while the false evaporates and the Gold Elixir immediately crystalizes."[5] As you undo the knots and adhesions that bind falsehood a new truthful reality emerges. The premise is that your truth is based on your own personal psychophysical energies—on the thoughts that arise and the directions they take. It is not based on a truth external to yourself. Once you gain this truth then internal power is unleashed, manifesting initially as inner healing and later resulting in the healing of the community.

Unfortunately there are many aspects of our society that cultivate fragmentation and loss of the truth. Fragmentation according to the classics is caused by fame, fortune, and indulgence in the external senses. Kan and Li practice reverses this trend and encourages a realignment of personal values through the firing and purification process. Liu reminds us again with, "One should take the opening to get to work, intensely refining them [water and fire] to burn away conditional temperament."[6] Once we align our personal values with our psychophysical energies, our own truth can emerge.

The goal of realigning our personal values to something that is sustaining is not unique to Taosim. According to the Koran (al-Baqarah 2:156), "Surely we belong to God and to Him shall we return." Buddhists seek to uncover the veil of Samsara and get off the wheel of misguided purpose to return to the emptiness of Nirvana. In the Tao, our purpose is to find the Wu Wei and join with the Tao. Perhaps all of these mystic traditions are saying the same thing. Therefore those who have an affinity with the Taoist path will realize that they are not alone and that other religions also propose the same objectives. The methods may be different but the goal is the same. As William Blake would say, "All religions are one."[7] This reassures the adept that his truth and reason for practice are not exceptional—rather, they are universal.

# IMMORTALITY

Most traditional Taoists would say the aim of Kan and Li practice is to become "immortal." Yet this term has so many layers and variations of meaning that it doesn't help most junior adepts. This is partly because ancient practices have become shrouded in myths and legends.

A common definition of immortality is the ability to live forever. This can occur at a physical or spiritual level. Another common understanding is that life continues after death. Still others regard immortality as being remembered long after your death. Some feel that if you leave behind offspring or notable deeds, then you and your name are consequently immortal. A more difficult concept to understand is "immortal consciousness," whereby the future and the past are experienced in one moment. Wittgenstein gives us an idea of this concept with, "If by eternity is understood not endless temporal duration but timelessness, then he lives eternally who lives in the present."[8]

In the Taoist framework, immortality has a few different meanings, which are discussed below.

## Ge Hong's Three Levels of Immortals

Ge Hong posited three levels of immortal existence: the simulated corpse, the earthbound transcendant, and the celestial transcendant.[9]

### *Simulated Corpse Mimicking Death*

In this form of immortality, the adept simulates death and is buried. However, he rises again as a physical being and escapes to live an unknown life of isolation.

This model has two levels of interpretation. The first is that the practitioner simulates death through meditation and medicines. In this quasi-dead state he is buried and then escapes from the coffin or tomb to live in the mountains. His achievement in this scenario is the giving up of community life to be at one with nature and the Tao. This was regarded as the lowest level of achievement, but the giving up of attachments—such as one's name and society status—are notable achievements that signify a deep commitment on behalf of the adept.

An alternate understanding is that the adept escapes in spirit form but the body disappears. This is close to the story of Jesus Christ[10] and represents a considerable achievement. These immortals have the ability to visit people in need either through visions or dreams. They are able to have a continual positive effect on the community after their alleged death.

### The Earthbound Transcendent

The earthly or middle level is where adepts can exist in the earthly realm for hundreds of years (again, usually in the mountains). They have the ability to appear in multiple places at the same time, and at various different times through history. This is regarded as a middle level immortal. The immortal Chan San-Feng apparently did this. Consequently, historians have long been confused as to when and where he actually lived.

### The Celestial Transcendant

Celestial immortals supposedly ascend to the void and join a pantheon of gods much like our own hierarchical bureaucratic society. Union with the void is a theme that transcends legend and miracles. Even though it is regarded as the highest level, it is theoretically very achievable for today's students: expansion of consciousness beyond self to the vast void and being lost in the moment equate with this experience. This theme will be revisited again and again throughout this text.

## Five Classes of Immortality According to Immortals Chung Li-Chuan and Lu Dong-Pin

Chung Li-Chuan and Lu Dong-Pin's five levels of immortality include ghosts, travelers on the lesser, middle, and great paths, and celestial immortals.[11]

### Ghost

This level results from poor practice whereby the adept engages the psychic realm without engaging the body. These ghosts have no name and are regarded as yin beings, unlike successful immortals, who are regarded as yang beings. All is not lost, however, as these ghosts can choose to enter the human realm again!

## The Lesser Path

Immortals on the Lesser Path remain in the human realm through a long life. They have strong bodies and are able to ward off disease. They understand Lu's teachings: "If you want to cultivate longevity then you first must refine the body so that you can survive the kalpas (karmic catastrophes) in the earthly realm."[12] Lesser Path immortals practice the "ten abstinences"[13]—refraining from grains, meat, thinking, sexual activity, physical labor, and talking and mixing with society, while cultivating breath control, saliva practice, and stillness.[14]

At this level there is a sense of self-denial, but it is not to be denigrated. The adept's prior existence or karma may have been so perverted that this ascetic existence is needed. However, progress to the next stage requires letting go to nature and becoming natural.

Lesser Path practitioners are concerned with "strengthening the lower tan tien,"[15] hence their practice correlates best with Lesser Kan and Li meditation. They are successful in their practice and are able to mate the dragon and tiger and form the immortal fetus.

The majority of serious UHT students are negotiating this realm. Many are confined to city life, teaching but allotting time for retreats and periods of a reclusive life.

## The Middle Path

Adepts on the Middle Path become "earth immortals," sitting halfway between the celestial and earthly realms. They understand the cycles of the seasons and the effects of the solar system on our planet, and are able to harmonize with these larger forces.

This practitioner has successfully engaged the practice of Kan and Li with specific focus on the Waterwheel and refining the elixir. She has completely opened the middle tan tien. Therefore this path corresponds best with the practices of Greater and Greatest Kan and Li.

### The Great Path

The Great Path indicates an adept who has successfully entered the spirit realm (fig. 2.4). He or she has fully gestated the immortal fetus and formed the spiritual body. Lu says of this spiritual body: "If you want to transcend the mundane and enter the sacred, you must refine the body and transmute it into vapor and then use your own body to create another body."[16] Following formation of the spiritual body, the successful adept is competent in prolonged periods of astral travel.

Ge Hong describes the Great Path in this way: "When the aspirant is accomplished, he will ride on the white crane and the scaled dragon to pay respects to the Immortal Ruler in the Supreme Void. There he will be given the decorated diploma which entitles him to the name of a Chen-jen (True Man)."[17]

In this travel, adepts are able to merge with the void,[18] thus obliterating self, time, and space (see fig. 2.5 on page 44). This void is difficult to place into words. However, we gain a glimpse through Lu Dong-Pin's teachings:

> When one is so far advanced that every shadow and every echo has disappeared, so that one is entirely quiet and firm, this is refuge within the cage of energy, when all that is miraculous returns to its roots. One does not alter the place, but the place divides itself. This is incorporeal space where a thousand and ten thousand places are one place. One does not alter the time, but the time divides itself. This is immeasurable time when all the aeons are like a moment.[19]

The Great Path best correlates with the ability to fully open the upper tan tien and therefore corresponds to the practice of Sealing of the Five Senses. Lu Dong-Pin says, "If you merge the spirit with the Tao and return it to the upper tan tien then you will be liberated from the mundane."[20]

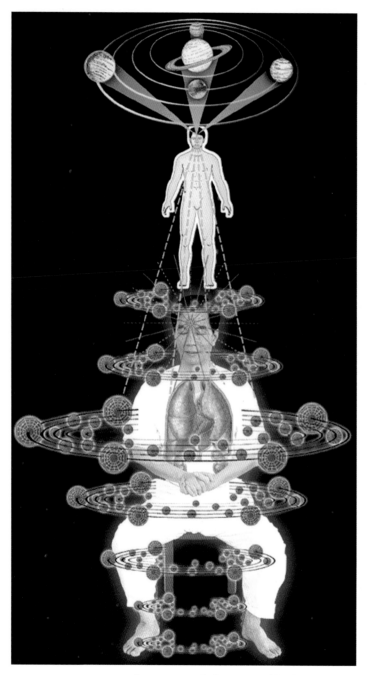

Fig. 2.4. On the Great Path the spiritual body
is fully formed.

Fig. 2.5. Time, space, and the observer
can merge into One.

### Celestial Immortal

Celestial immortality is the highest level of immortal achievement (fig. 2.6). Here the practitioner ascends (possibly in broad daylight and visible to others),[21] and the body is left as a pile of dust with perhaps only nails, hair, or even a pearl remaining. Ge Hong documented many adepts who successfully attained this level, including Chen An-Shi, Yin Chang-Sheng, Hua Zi-Qi, and Wu Mu.[22]

These immortals gain the right to sit in the pantheon of Taoist deities and partake in leadership of the earthly realm. This practice probably

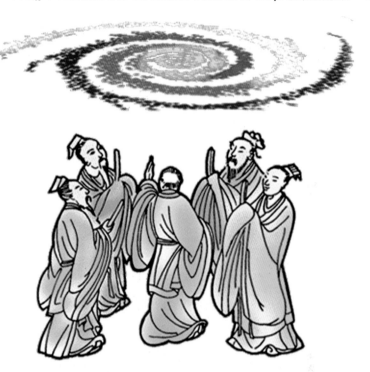

Fig. 2.6. Celestial immortals earn the right to sit in
the pantheon of Taoist deities.

best correlates with the Congress of Heaven and Earth and the Reunion
of Heaven and Man.

Embarking on the path to Kan and Li practice clearly involves a
commitment beyond the ordinary. It belongs to those who sincerely
seek immortality on some level. At the very least, the practice compels
us to realize the kind of immortality inherent in perceiving the unitive
state. Once the adept has glimpsed this void—known also as the One,
the nothingness, the Wu Wei, and enlightenment—he has touched
immortality. This level of immortality is readily achievable by the
reader.

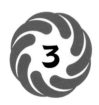

# Principles of the Greatest Kan and Li Meditation

*When you understand nothingness that is nothing. Then in preserving oneness you'll know there is no One. When One and Nothing are both overturned, the great task of nothingness and oneness is done.*

LI DAO-CHUN[1]

The fundamental principles of Kan and Li meditation were presented in detail in *The Practice of Greater Kan and Li.* This volume continues those discussions with the purpose of taking the reader to an even higher level of understanding of the doctrine surrounding the Greatest Kan and Li meditation.

# MYSTIC PHILOSOPHY

## The Growth of the Spiritual Infant

*The mind is like the full moon shining deep in the night,*
*its light pervading above and below, heaven and earth;*
*the gold elixir crystallizes in the great void of space.*

LIU I-MING[2]

There are several ways of describing the adept's stages of development in Kan and Li practice. Most of the terminology comes from a mix of sexual and External Alchemy metaphors. The External Alchemy framework was the first model for describing the fragmented parts and also for defining the goal of the practice. In the language of External Alchemy, the goal is the Medicine or the Golden Elixir that provides everlasting life.

The sexual metaphor is a description of the techniques that are specific to Internal Alchemy; it has become the dominant model of Kan and Li practice. In Inner Alchemy, sexual desire is the driving force for the union of the disparate parts of self into one. The One is born as the spiritual infant that can reunite with Heaven and Earth and achieve immortal status.

The sexual metaphor can be extended to describe the meditation's increasing levels of complexity as the conception, gestation, birth, and nurturing of the spiritual infant. In this framework, the stages include:

1. Gathering the Primordial Force
2. Conception
3. Embryo
4. Completing gestation and the Lesser Medicine
5. Birth of the spiritual infant
6. Breast-feeding

7. Spiritual body and ecstatic flight
8. Education of the spiritual child
9. Return home

Before continuing this discussion, we must stress that the sexual basis of this mystical path is *just a metaphor*. The metaphor helps describe the ephemeral feelings and forces that drive the process. They are not to be used as guidelines for visualization. The embryo is not to be visualized as an actual fetus, for instance: it is a dense experience of the primordial nothingness. We will continue to emphasize this point throughout the text, as it is an important one for practitioners to understand.

## Gathering the Primordial Force

Students first experience the Primordial Force in the Microcosmic Orbit and Three Tan Tiens practices. In the Microcosmic Orbit, there is a gathering of energies from the major acupuncture points in the Governor and Conception vessels along with the earthly, heavenly, and cosmic forces. In the Three Tan Tiens practice, the energies of the Crystal Palace, the heart, and the lower tan tien are brought together. In both meditations, the various energies are all congealed into a vague nondescript vapor or essence in the lower tan tien.

Fusion practices are the next step. They blend the five elemental forces using spiraling techniques and sexual energy to create the pearl. This time the sense of the primordial is both thicker and deeper. Note that although this force is called a "pearl," each student is different, and each experience is different than the ones before it: the student should not become attached to particular words or descriptions. Furthermore, the different terms appear with much variation and inconsistency in the Taoist literature. They can be used to describe the beginner's experience as well as the most advanced practitioner's description of the Golden Elixir.

## Conception

Conception occurs when the primordial force is inseminated with orgasm power in Fusion, Lesser Kan and Li, or Greater Kan and Li practice. During Fusion, if the student has a real sense of the primordial and accompanies this with orgasm, then conception can occur. In Lesser Kan and Li, conception occurs with ejaculation and insemination of the essence of the liver spirit (Hun). Similarly in Greater Kan and Li, there is orgasm and insemination of the spleen spirit (Yi).

## Embryo

The embryo is usually *not* experienced as an inner physical fetus with arms and legs! If this is happening, the student may be visualizing too much rather than merging all the inner senses. The embryo is a symbol. It is sensed as a deep Primordial Chi that merges the inner with the outer, the past and the future, and identity of the whole with one's self. To this point Liu I-Ming says, "the spiritual embryo is formless and immaterial; though it is called an embryo, in reality no embryo is to be seen. The term embryo just describes true awareness becoming stabilized, not scattering."[3]

Liu I-Ming further describes this state in the womb as an empty circle: "The ultimate of non-being; no shape, no form; (and) no sound, no smell."[4] This state of mind is also a feature of other mystical traditions. When a Buddhist describes "emptiness" and a Christian uses the term "God," they are likely to be describing the same mystical experience.

## Completing Gestation
## and the Lesser Medicine

The embryo requires ten months of incubation. This time period is somewhat arbitrary but is set to match the reality of the physical realm.[5]

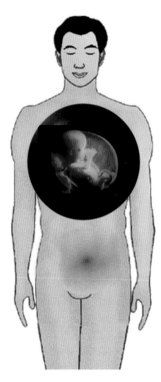

Fig. 3.1. Though it may help the beginning student to view the spiritual embryo as a physical fetus, as shown here, advanced students know that the embryo is formless. It is an experience of true awareness becoming stabilized.

This incubation time is called *lien hsu ho Tao.*[6] Like an actual pregnancy, a spiritual pregnancy can be lost as a result of physical illness or stress. Most importantly, the work that the student performed in creating the conception must be maintained for a prolonged period without interruptions.

The pregnancy is cultivated largely in the lower tan tien. This is because it needs the nurturing aspect of the earth—the clay cauldron—rather than the harshness of iron (solar plexus) or jade (heart). The clay cauldron is symbolically connected to the earth. It is caring like a loving mother. Liu I-Ming reinforces this principle when he states, "The medicine going back in the earth pot is a symbol for the work of incubation, gentle nurturance, of the spiritual embryo formed by the joining of yin and yang."[7]

For most adepts, gestation means continual practice for most of the day for a period of many months. However, who is to say that episodic practice while mingling with city life won't work? We are in a new stage of evolution of Taoist practice. Now Westerners are openly taught these practices in a systematic and well thought-out manner. Perhaps multiple short-term episodes of practice over some years could also produce the same achievement! The nurturing required to complete the pregnancy will be discussed further in chapter 8.

In the UHT system there is a stage of development in the gestational period called the Lesser Medicine. This term describes the stage of practice when the embryo merges with the Greater Spirit and facilitates the complete merging of all the adept's inner spirits. In particular, it marks the merging of the higher Shen from the brain with the other inner spirits. The adept may experience this Lesser Medicine as a profound yet vague essence of the primordial. Other students experience it as something more solid. Similarly, Liu I-Ming describes it as a "bead," saying, "The primordial energy comes from nothingness and crystallizes into a black bead, the spiritual embryo takes on form."[8] This solid "form" may be the reason for also calling this stage the "Lesser Pill"—as the pill connotes something hard. In Fusion practice we referred to this condensation as a "pearl."

Coupling in the heart involves the lower Shen as well. The experience of seeing the light of the Greater Spirit humbles the higher Shen in the brain into an attitude of self-sacrifice. No longer seeing itself "above" the other spirits, the higher Shen becomes willing to merge with the others in the embryo. With an ambience of serving the greater good, the higher Shen fuses with the others. The Greater Spirit manifests as a powerful light or vortex and could be the Celestial Emperor or the Cinnabar Sovereign. The formula Gathering the Lesser Medicine in chapter 6 is specific for marking this stage.

### Commentary on the Lesser Medicine

In this formation of the Lesser Medicine there are a few concepts worth enumerating. *Medicine* is a term frequently used in translations of Taoist Inner Alchemical practice. However, associated terms such as *pill* and *elixir* are also used. It is uncertain whether the author and translator imply any difference in the alchemical meanings of these different words. My supposition (Andrew Jan) is that they can be used interchangeably.

The purpose of the medicine or elixir for the Taoist was to heal the body, promote longevity, and ultimately to produce immortality. The embryo and the medicine are of the same stuff. It is probably just a question of grade and quality. To begin with, the merging of the three tan tiens is a medicine in itself. Liu I-Ming defines "effective medicine" as the "primordial true, unified energy; it is primordial vitality, energy and spirit, the three treasures."[9] Liu goes on to explain that the gathering of these three energies of the upper, middle, and lower tan tiens is akin to the transmissions from the Three Pure Ones. Then the adept uses the alchemical fire to merge them into one.

The next stage, as Chang Po-Tuan defines it, is one where "the Medicines are produced in the occult opening . . . when the dragon and tiger have mated."[10] A higher quality energy is produced after a significant gestation period whereby the embryo has joined and experienced the essence and spirits of the three tan tiens. The Lesser Medicine is formed when the higher Shen and Greater Spirit merge into the embryo.

Alchemists such as Chang San-Feng try to distinguish the medicine from the embryo. Chang says, "When Spirit enters energy, it forms an embryo; when energy cleaves to spirit, it crystalizes the alchemical pill."[11] Evidently the alchemical pill doesn't just need for the spirit to enter; the spirit must also stay and cleave (adhere strongly) for months! The Greater Medicine is thus both a higher-grade formulation and one left to mature for longer. So now the adept can "return to the origin, arise from death and restore life, preserve and make the body complete, becoming master of the great medicine."[12]

For the Greater Spirit to fuse with the inner spirits, the powers of mindfulness, love, and orgasm are required. Mindfulness is required to respect the philosophy and spiritual hierarchy involved in such a union. Love is required to create the softness, delicateness, and cherishing required for such an event. Orgasm calls upon the creation power of the universe to seal it permanently.

Some readers may better understand the process of merging with the Greater Spirit and birth of the spiritual infant through the teachings of Jesus Christ. This spiritual birth is described in John 3:3 of the King James Bible:

> Jesus answered and said unto him, "Verily, verily, I say unto thee, except a man be born again, he cannot see the kingdom of God." Nicodemus saith unto him, "How can a man be born when he is old? Can he enter the second time into his mother's womb, and be born?" Jesus answered, "Verily, verily, I say unto thee, except a man be born of water and of the Spirit, he cannot enter into the kingdom of God. That which is born of the flesh is flesh; and that which is born of the spirit is spirit. Marvel not that I said unto thee, Ye must be born again!"

In the Christian tradition, the Greater Spirit is the Holy Spirit, often described as white light resembling the fluttering, lightness, and purity of a dove. Interpreting the line "born of water and of the Spirit" from a Kan and Li perspective would say that Li is formed by the delicate heavenly fire of spirit and water from the sexual power of the earth. Once this union is achieved and the spiritual embryo has completed its gestation, the adept is ready to be reborn.

## Birth of the Spiritual Infant

The actual birth of the spiritual infant may be a continuation of the above event or may occur on a separate occasion. Here, the Greater Spirit returns again, indicating that the embryo is now complete and ready to be born to an independent existence. This union of the Greater Spirit with the embryo enables transmutation of the fetus. Hence, "the emergence of the infant means the release and the transmutation of the spiritual embryo."[13] This birth indicates success in having formed the Golden Elixir (Golden Flower). Again, the student should not be distracted by such terms. Li Dao-Chun, a master alchemist and prolific writer of the twelfth to thirteenth centuries, says:

> Gold Elixir is just a name—how could it have form? That it is visible does not mean it can be seen with the eyes. . . . You can hardly call it non-existent, but when you look at it you cannot see it, and when you grasp it you cannot comprehend it, so you can hardly call it existent.[14]

The spiritual infant or Golden Elixir is really just a solid experience of empty space or nothingness, though some describe it as something physically solid. They say, "Because the Gold Elixir pill is round and bright, it is represented as a pearl; because its spiritual subtlety is hard to express, it is also represented as a mystic pearl."[15] If we realize the difficulties of describing mystical experience, then it is much easier to understand how all the meditation-based traditions can be talking about the same experience. Certainly the Taoist rebirth would be described in Buddhism as equivalent to attaining complete awakening or "the wish-fulfilling gem."[16] In Christian mysticism, "rebirth" or the formation of the philosopher's stone represents this same achievement. Hinduism (and Taoism) use the term *enlightenment* to describe this experience. Ultimate realization is to merge consciousness with God. God is that deep experience of both nothing and everything.

The reader may be confused and this is understandable: we are trying to find words for the indescribable. The unitive state has so many names and symbols, ranging from pearls and stones to elixirs and medicines, from embryos to spiritual bodies, from nothingness to enlightenment, and finally from emptiness to Oneness. Furthermore, the stages of completion also overlap at this level. It is somewhat artificial to attempt to separate them chronologically or by levels of complexity. Nevertheless, the attempt is worthwhile. We just ask the reader to recognize the difficulty of the teacher's task in verbalizing the desired stages and achievements.

### *Womb Breathing*

Rebirth is also marked by the onset of Womb Breathing, an involuntary indrawing and outdrawing of the abdomen without the movement of air through the upper or lower airways.[17] Commentary on the *Triplex Unity* says, "Practical refinement must reach Womb Breathing before energy returns to the ocean of the fundamental; this is the process of gestation."[18] Because of this observation, some masters designate Womb Breathing as a fundamental achievement.

Although it starts in the abdomen, Womb Breathing can eventually involve the entire body, and it may be associated with swallowing saliva and chi. It is extremely pleasant. The whole body feels soft, fluid, and connected. If there is any remaining tension in the body, then this Womb Breathing will surely remove it. The experience further opens the body and prepares the spiritual birth canal (Central Thrusting Channel) for the release of the spiritual body.

## Breast-Feeding

Just when you thought that all the work was done! Unfortunately the process of perfection continues. While glimpses of the Wu Wei have been wonderful, there are still more challenges ahead. Chang Po-Tuan describes this current stage as "enlightened but not shining."[19]

Once the infant has been born, there is a transition period in which the infant can freely move up and down through the various cauldron levels and travel for short distances from the crown. In the chest (corresponding to the cauldron site of Greatest Kan and Li), the phenomenon of spiritual breast-feeding occurs.[20]

In terms of spiritual practice, there may be prolonged periods of cessation of external breathing with swallowing of saliva and chi. This Elixir Chi Kung mimics breast-feeding. Therefore the adept should reproduce the mind-set of a suckling infant, feeling loved, bonded, and sustained. Breast-feeding includes some sexual feeling for both the mother and infant, so please give yourself permission for some sexual arousal. Likewise the monkey mind turns itself off and retreats into some pleasant state of feeling whole.

The gentle suckling that occurs at this depth of meditation can synchronize with the craniosacral pump and replace the external breath. This profound depth removes all deep traumas and negative societal conditioning from the body.[21]

The duration of this stage, according to the classics, is three years. This may have been the time that mothers suckled their children. In our society the World Health Organization recommends around eighteen months.

In *Twenty-Four Secrets,* Chang says that during these three years "real consciousness is refined into a golden body. Knowing before and after, the sage is spiritual."[22]

## Spiritual Body and Ecstatic Flight

Now that the adept has nurtured the spiritual infant, a spiritual body (Golden Body) is formed by transferring the immaterial essence of the physical body up into the energy body to give it form. This can require a detailed connection to every physical part of the body, including acupuncture channels and the tan tiens. In this connection, the essence or imprint of each physical form is made light and raised up into the energy body. This whole process can then be repeated to create another body on top of the energy body—two body-lengths above the crown. This work requires profoundly deep meditation and the ability to work with very purified energies. These energies are the spirits of the organs in their most fundamental form, appearing now as delicate translucent vortices rather than the thicker and heavier energetic forms.

At this stage, an excursion into outer space is easy. Liu I-Ming says: "When the cluster of mundanity has been stripped away, the embryo fully developed, the elixir is done; like a ripe melon dropping off the vine, one suddenly breaks through the undifferentiated, bursts out with pure spiritual body, leaps into the realm of absolute open nothingness and transcends the world."[23] With practice, the adept can travel outside of the physical body for longer and longer periods of time.

### Physical Ascension

The process of forming the spiritual body is similar to the mechanism of physical ascension, the technique Ge Hong refers to as "ascension in broad daylight." The actual details of this method are beyond the scope of this text, but the principle involves making the essence of each organ—including flesh and bones—so light and pure that they rise up to the immortal body. At this level of purity and lightness, the material transforms into the immaterial. Ge Hong documented the names and methods of many immortals that achieved this feat.[24] In the Christian tradition, Elijah and Moses also accomplished this level.

## Educating the Original Spirit

The Original Spirit—the merged team of nine inner spirits—is educated at a very subtle level. It "learns" as the adept connects to planetary and stellar bodies. These heavenly objects are absorbed and digested while the spirit travels out of the body. Journeying far out into the universe, the adept can pass through wormholes to reach distant locations. The further she travels, the purer the energy she encounters. At times, dark matter can seem like a refined elixir. Using another metaphor, education can be considered like gathering high-octane fuel. The more refined the energy, the more powerful it becomes.

## Return Home

For many Taoist practitioners, returning to their original birth star is an important goal. This is a major event, which may be the end of the road for some, or a stopover for more daring travelers.

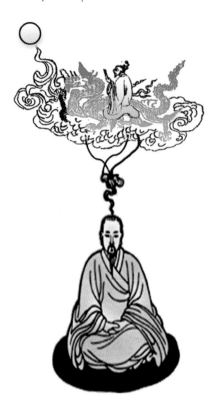

Fig. 3.2. The return home
is a return to the Source.

With further flight, the adept has little or no thought and is captured by the bliss of space travel. In this realm, time is not linear. Eventually, the adept forgets the past and the future and dwells for prolonged periods in the moment. Time stands still, and the adept comprehends one of the three important aspects of immortality.

In this timeless state, the nature of space alters as well: the immense distances and geography of the universe can be both comprehended and navigated. This enables the adept to begin to condense the universe into "nothingness." Chang Po-Tuan describes this as "Appearing, hiding, going against or along, no one can fathom it . . . the universe is ultimately empty."[25]

According to Chang Po-Tuan, the great masters would remain in this stage of development for nine years. However, once over this "wall,"[26] the adept lets go completely, and time, space, and observership dissolve. There is now complete reunion with the Tao.

From there the adept is reborn yet again. The immortal now takes on a role within the celestial immortal hierarchy, to oversee humanity and all living creatures on Earth.

## THE STAGES OF THE EMBRYO DEVELOPMENT AND CORRESPONDING UHT FORMULAS

| STAGE | EXPERIENCE | FORMULA |
|---|---|---|
| 1. Gathering the Primordial Force | Pleasant, smooth, sea of chi in lower tan tien; denser experience described as a pearl | Microcosmic Orbit and Fusion practice |
| 2. Conception | Five elemental energies fused with orgasm energy; Kan and Li energies coupled and inseminated by organ spirits | Fusion, Lesser Kan and Li |
| 3. Embryo | Nourishing, further growth and further insemination of body's inner spirits | Lesser, Greater, and Greatest Kan and Li, and Sealing of the Five Senses |
| 4. Completing gestation/ Lesser Medicine | Final insemination of the Higher Shen as the last inner spirit along with the Greater Spirit | Greatest Kan and Li |
| 5. Birth of the spiritual infant/Greater Medicine | Insemination of Greater Spirit and onset of Womb Breathing | Greatest Kan and Li |
| 6. Breast-feeding | Infant rests on heart tan tien accompanied by swallowing chi | Greatest Kan and Li and Sealing of the Five Senses |
| 7. Spiritual body and ecstatic flight | Developed spiritual body; swallowing Chi and flight through outer space | Lesser, Greater, Greatest Kan and Li, and Sealing of the Five Senses |
| 8. Education of the spiritual child | Absorption of planetary, stellar, and dark matter energies | Greatest Kan and Li and Sealing of the Five Senses |
| 9. Return home | Return to birth star then dissolution of self into Wu Wei | Congress of Heaven and Earth, Reunion of Heaven and Man |

# METHODOLOGY

The main methods of Taoist Inner Alchemy derive from the concepts and practices of External Alchemy, sexuality, cooking, and Taoist creation theory.

## External Alchemy

In *The Practice of Greater Kan and Li,* we explained how External Alchemists used a dual mixture of cinnabar and lead, firing these to produce mercury (grease of dragons) and silver (true essence of tiger).* These last two elements are finally combined to produce the Golden Elixir. Upon ingestion, this elixir would supposedly confer immortal life.

In Kan and Li practice, Kan is associated with lead. Upon purifying Kan ☵ we distill pure yang as pure Heaven ☰. Upon purifying Li ☲ we end up with pure yin presented as the trigram Earth ☷. When Earth is placed submissively above Heaven ䷊ it gradually transforms into the unitive state ☰. This unitive state correlates with the Primordial Chi and is the origin of alchemical medicine and the spiritual fetus.

Dragon Gate Taoism expands these alchemical metaphors to explain the development of consciousness, which is a helpful concept for UHT practice. True Lead correlates with silver and the inner tiger's vigor (pure yang). It embodies the principles of firmness and gravity. In terms of mind, True Lead represents true knowledge. True Mercury, on the other hand, is more yin as it is mutable like water. It represents flexible consciousness and spiritual essence.

The initial aim of Kan and Li practice is to remove false knowledge from the mind. False knowledge is information that promotes separation and fragmentation of the souls and spirits within the body. In some respects, this is a kind of tautology that doesn't really help the practitioner grasp the meaning of the steps in mind transformation. It is rather

---

*The metaphors of the tiger and the dragon will be discussed in detail later in this chapter.

like saying, "what gets you to the merged state is what gets you to the merged state!" Nevertheless, with some lateral thought, the practitioner can see that knowledge that makes us arrogant, proud, or that fosters separation is by definition classified as false knowledge.

## Cooking

The concept of cooking as a metaphysical practice was first introduced in External Alchemy. Preparation of the elixir was a delicate and prolonged process whereby toxic heavy metal oxides were "cooked according to cosmic instructions and surrounded by magical devices."[27] The use of fire, water, and various other ingredients has obvious parallels to the art of cooking food. Special ingredients ranged from blood and animal products to oyster shells and sea salt. There is an overlap here between preparation of healing herbs and magical practice. The parts of animals and humans would confer special spiritual powers depending on the character and nature of the donor.

In the cooking of food, fire and water are central to the preparation, breakdown, and mixing of foodstuffs to create something that is both digestible and palatable for human consumption. In Internal Alchemy, "Purification and cooking are carried out by the fire or by water."[28]

In Fusion practice, the elemental energies from the five organs become the various flavors that make up a special soup. This special soup has two predominant forms: it can make a primordial broth or alternatively a compassion brew.

In Kan and Li practice, Water Chi from the kidneys is initially heated by heart and adrenal fire. Later, the organs are steam-cooked in such a way that their yin essence can be withdrawn and placed again in the cooking pot (cauldron). Different types of cooking occur at the various cauldron levels. In the clay pot in the lower tan tien, we have a low-to-moderate broad-based heat that is meant for slow cooking. It is suitable for preparing a primordial essence that will become a fetus. The solar plexus tan tien is made from iron and can take a stronger fire and stronger yang emotions. The heart tan tien's cauldron is made of jade and cannot take a strong heat at all. It requires distant fire and steam to avoid cracking it. Yet its essence is exquisite like love. Likewise in the Sealing of the Five Senses, we have a cauldron in the Crystal Palace or on the tip of the nose; it requires an even more delicate heat. Chang Po-Tuan reminds us that without delicate cooking and the ability to use various temperatures according to the coarseness of our brew, we will not achieve our goal. He says, "Gentle cooking and fierce refinement are the methods of immortals."[29]

Furthermore, the duration of the cooking process is key to success. "Knowing when to apply fast and slow fires is crucial in Internal Alchemy," Eva Wong reminds us.[30] Blindly intense continuous firing in the cauldrons will not achieve the desired result; on the contrary, there need to be rest periods from the cooking process.

### Regulating the Fire

In *The Practice of Greater Kan and Li* we discussed various ways of regulating the fire and the role of the attendant. Regulating the fire can involve hastening it by "fanning it," or reducing it, which is sometimes achieved by placing the tiger (inner fire) in the ocean. At times, the attendant might even turn off the fire (Chao Pi-Chen calls this "freezing the fire"[31]), in order to allow other vital processes to occur. These might include gathering energies from space travel, dealing with a discovered blockage, making an intellectual realization, or digesting the essence you've made.

## Taoist Creation Theory

The process of reducing multiplicity to unity is essentially a reversal of the Taoist creation or cosmological theory, wherein the One becomes many. In order to find the One, the body's individual elements need to be identified and merged. This merging is a vital process by which mystical consciousness is achieved.

The pakua is used in conjunction with this process. The pakua is an eight-sided symbol that has representations of the five elements (two for water) with Heaven and Earth (making eight forces). (See fig. 3.3.) The center is composed of the Tai Chi symbol, which includes yin and yang entwining. The eight forces correspond to the eight immortals, who have completed the alchemical process and realized mystical consciousness.[32]

Sexual energy is a force that brings opposites together and creates

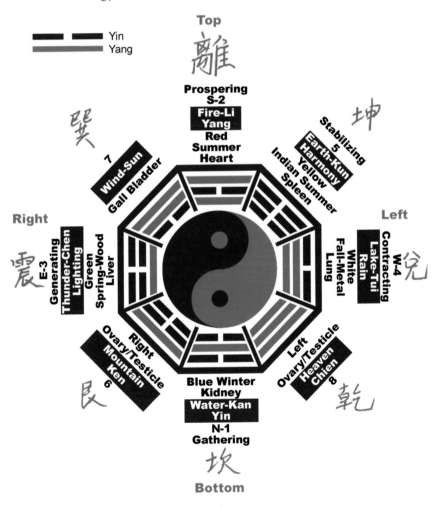

Fig. 3.3. The pakua: eight forces condensing
into a duality of yin and yang

something new: it contributes special uniting power that can fuse the seemingly disparate energies of the elements. Once discovered, the five elements can be reduced to a duality of Kan and Li or yin and yang. Sexual energy is used to resolve this duality with one final coupling.[33] In Kan and Li, the merging of this duality brings us closer to forming the embryo and the Golden Elixir. Sensing the Original Chi as an embryo is equivalent to sensing the unitive state of the Tao.[34]

## No Method

"No Method" describes the principle of letting go, which is vital to the experience of the One. The following story highlights the importance of no method.

> Once upon a time in ancient China there was a famous Taoist master. He had inspired so many students with his calm demeanor and loving heart. He was reputed to have the ability to vaporize into thin air and to appear in multiple places at the same time. There was a young man called Xiao Wei who was besotted by this master. Xiao Wei made his way through the adoring crowds until he was standing face to face with the legendary man.
>
> He asked, "What do I need to do to become as you are?" To his surprise, the immortal said, "See that mountain over there? Find yourself a cave, sit in it, and do nothing for thirty years." The adept was shocked. He was expecting a hundred secret Inner Alchemical formulas or maybe a list of concoctions of metals to distill, fuse, and ingest. Such a statement shocked him to the core.
>
> He looked inside himself and asked a question to his deepest aspect of his being. "This is too simple; could it be true?" Off Xiao Wei went to the mountains. He sat and he sat and he sat. Occasionally he would eat a little food (some nuts and roots) and practice some Chi Kung taught to him by other masters.

After five years, he started to have some doubts. "Was the master's advice true?" Maybe what the master told him was a way to get rid of him. However, Xiao Wei did notice many changes within himself. He delighted in his quietude and the delicate worlds that had already been exposed to him. He decided to try a little longer.

After ten years, he had progressed in his practice. He could leave his body and begin to unite with Heaven and Earth, but he became afraid when he thought he would die in this merging. His doubt grew, so he went outside the cave, and then noticed that a whole town was built around the foot of the mountain, with his name written in front of all the temples. This frightened and confused him. He decided to retreat back to his cave for some peace and solitude.

After thirty years, he had learned to merge with Heaven and Earth. What he had previously known of himself had been forgotten. He had developed a wonderful compassion for all living creatures. He believed that he and the universe are one! He came down to the village and crowds gathered! He realized now that the whole town was dedicated to him.* The lead abbot came up to him and asked what the details of his practice were.

He told them, "Sit and do nothing for thirty years and all shall be revealed!" To this the chief abbot turned his back in disgust. Soon the townspeople abandoned their dedication and most of the inhabitants decided to move on. Xiao Wei stared and contemplated those who were still left. He could hold on no longer and at that instant he let go. His flesh disappeared in a puff of smoke and ascended. He became immortal and will live as long as Heaven and Earth.

The principle of this story is meant to provide the reader with the counter position for this entire text. Within this book are a multitude

---

*There is a temple in Xian named after an immortal who achieved transcendence by "doing nothing."

of formulas. Given the parable above, what should the reader do? We are not advising the reader to ignore the formulas but to understand deeply that discovery of the Tao is a natural process of returning to the "uncarved block." The formulas assist the adept in unwinding back to the core but are not the endpoint in themselves. Formulas come and go and change—not only within a sect, but also between sects and different mystical traditions. They are meant for contemplation and dialogue, not as laws written in stone. Each person is different with varied issues and lessons. Each meditation sitting is unique and should be treated on its merits.

The formulas provide lessons, which do need to be mastered. In the parable above, the master may have spent thirty years learning methods and techniques before he was ready to do "nothing." The formulas help us align with the principle of apophasis—the principle of undoing rather than doing. Each of us has been a fetus before, so each of us theoretically just has to let go of temporal conditioning and return. The formulas merely assist us in this unwinding process. Like many skills, the formulas can be seemingly forgotten once they have been mastered and integrated.

In our experience most Westerners try too hard and do too much. This is the dark aspect of our Western culture. Because the student expects and does too much, the body and mind cannot fully relax. Consequently, the adept fails to achieve the required internal experiences and gives up. Again, the aim is to undo and return.

However, the undoing should not be taken to the extreme of spiritual laziness. Liu I-Ming explains that if he carried "non-doing" to an extreme, the adept would just drown himself in passive "quietism."[35] The "doing," which is the formula aspects of Kan and Li, provides a counter to this doing nothing. Much like the principle of Kan and Li and the coupling of yin and yang, the coupling of doing and not doing is another duality. It is a blend and engagement of the two poles that creates the right balance of effort.

Achieving this state of mind is not difficult and is readily accessible to all. Remember we all came from this state as fetuses in the mother's womb; accessing it again requires nothing more than undoing and returning. This state of mind does not require performance of miracles. It doesn't require membership in a church or organization. It doesn't require death or a long life of suffering and hard labor in order to find it. These latter notions are all ways that religion has misinformed its followers in order to control them. Humanity and its perversion of religious doctrine have made access to this state of mind more and more difficult. The biggest lie is that only death will bring peace. What is the point of being in a blissful calm state if you're dead! It is likely that you won't even be conscious of it!

Therefore the advice for UHT students is to remember that the formulas provide a framework for the student to set up the process of undoing. In other words, the student lets go or falls into these formulas by relaxing and smiling. If the student contrives and manipulates too early then the coupling will not hold. The unwinding or letting go process allows the student to enter naturally into a formula.

Advanced students have learned many formulas in the course of their training. The best approach is to attempt to master each formula individually, which may involve repeat attendance at specific workshops and the assistance of audiovisual aids. Each meditation session will be different and the student will eventually allow one of many formulas taught over the years to arise spontaneously. This could include one of the Fusion formulas, or any of the formulas taught up to this point in the Kan and Li series. Bear the goal in mind—merging with the Tao—and allow the formulas to drop in to your meditation. Allow them to assist with the unwinding and returning to "nothing." Sometimes you may have to conjure up a missing link from your own experience—a practice that may not have been overtly taught by our system.

A student will often start with expectations and adhere to the prescribed formulas. Then at some stage in the meditation, he lets go and allows the energies or internal rhythms to take over. Once this threshold has been surpassed nothing else remains to be done. From here on the practitioner may only need to keep reminding himself to let go and enjoy the ride. This is particularly so when you begin to form the embryo. Here, the mind is captured by the blissful "unified energy."[36] No thoughts can arise and there is only passive following. This is the "non-doing" phase, which is essential to accessing the higher realms. Liu I-Ming says of this phase, "When you get to this state, doing is ended and non-doing appears; it is no longer necessary to strive—leave it to nature. It is like fruit growing on the branch—eventually they will ripen; the child in the belly will one day be born."[37]

Letting go also occurs in guided meditation as the student lets go to the teacher's guidance. However, the letting go of solo practice is more difficult, as expectations and distracting thoughts are seemingly stronger. Unlike in guided practice, students in solo meditation must learn to follow their own lead. Just like Push Hands, one follows the direction of the meditation and the lure that has the more powerful thread. It may be the breath, the pulse, deep pleasure in the Primordial Chi, merging, spiraling, or just the simple pleasure of dissolving. The formulas provide you with the skills to handle such varieties of meditation experience.

As soon as there is too much "doing," however, meditation becomes blocked. Too much doing includes excessive visualization. The move toward darkness and nothingness includes fusion of all the senses into one complete sensation of unity: do not get stuck in trying to see every color, every form, and every image. After many years of practice I (Andrew Jan) had moments where I thought my mind was changing for the worse. No longer did I see the bright colors of the organs in such practices as the Inner Smile. When I relaxed, my body would just melt away into "one dark night."*[38] Whereas colors may be important for the novice just learning to visualize, the precepts associated with beginner's practice should be forgotten by the advanced practitioner. Liu I-Ming believes that many adepts become misdirected by getting attached to visualizations instead of allowing the necessary merging of awareness with the nothingness of the Wu Wei![39]

---

*St. John of the Cross was a Christian mystic who wrote the poem *The Dark Night,* referring to the unitive experience.

Visualization is not wrong if it is integrated with the other senses. If you can hold on to a tactile sense of the yin essence in the cauldron—the formation of the primordial—while hearing the sounds of the tiger or dragon, then the visualization is both valid and empowering. However, students can easily get locked in the monkey mind and remain in the intellectual/visualization mode alone. The aim is to move toward a more holistic integrated state of awareness.

## INTERACTION BETWEEN THE FRAGMENTED PARTS

The principle of merging the fragmented parts, which is the essence of Kan and Li practice, can apply to many disparate categories of "parts." While many of these fragments were addressed in *The Practice of Greater Kan and Li,* this chapter is intended to add both breadth and depth to those discussions.

## I Ching Interpretation of Kan and Li Alchemical Practice

In *The Practice of Greater Kan and Li* we introduced the concept of Kan and Li collecting impure energies from the eight trigrams before the purification process could begin. The I Ching text offers deep insight into the nature of the Inner Alchemical work required in Kan and Li practice. These profound observations are largely provided by the work of Liu I-Ming and the wonderful translation by Thomas Cleary.[40] Liu offers us a foundation Taoist paradigm to realign our intention with our Kan and Li practice. His discussion is summarized below.

### *Returning to Heaven*

The ultimate goal of immortality is represented by the hexagram Heaven ☰. This represents a complete yang body, equivalent to the body of a deity. When an adept is successful at Kan and Li practice, he achieves this yang body.

When we are born, there is merging of pure yin and pure yang. Pure yin is represented by the hexagram Earth ䷁ and represents our material nature. Pure yang represents our spiritual nature. Together they rest in some momentary stillness, which can be symbolized by the hexagram Tranquillity: ䷊.

Unfortunately, incorrect conditioning by society, parents, and our own mistaken judgment causes our tranquil energies to scatter. Yang energies tend to rise while yin energies fall; the ultimate endpoint of this process is the hexagram Obstruction ䷋. The various hexagrams of the I Ching represent the journey of degradation toward this point of Obstruction, or the journey of redemption back toward Tranquillity ䷊ and then to Heaven ䷀.

The first step to salvation in our Kan and Li practice is to identify the energies of Kan ䷜ and Li ䷝. Kan represents our contaminated earthly nature, and is signified by the tiger. Kan is outwardly yin but inwardly yang ䷜. Li is our heavenly aspect polluted by our earthly desires. The dragon represents Li, which is outwardly yang but inwardly yin ䷝.

The next huge step is to stop the inevitable deterioration, effectively placing Kan above Li. This endeavor is the beginning of the "great work" and the basis of this entire text. Kan and Li practice occurs not only in meditation sessions, but ideally in all those other waking and sleeping moments in our lives as well. Kan and Li practice is the seed that eventually grows into the spiritual infant and finally returns home as the yang body. Our material and earthly life gradually transforms in front of our eyes as a reflection of this inner work.

## Misdirected Energies

Cleary and Liu offer the concepts of eliminating false yang and false yin energies. False yin refers to those yin energies such as misdirected love,

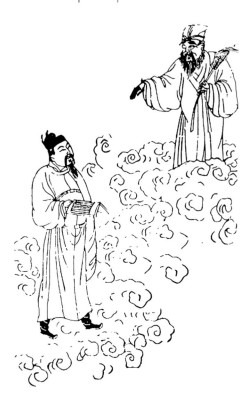

Fig. 3.4. Immortal Liu ascending to heaven after transforming his energies from the hexagram Tranquillity, making a totally yang body

inappropriate kindness, or false courage that take us toward fragmentation and death. Misdirected love may include love of entertainment and fine foods. False courage can see us doing silly things like making wars or acts of violence. False yang includes undue worry or anger. One can worry about one's reputation, be angry over material possessions, or impatient over one's practice.

I (Andrew Jan) have some issue with this principle of false energies. It is my belief that there are no false energies or desires. All energies are holy—some are just misdirected because of incorrect knowledge or intention. True knowledge takes us toward unity and immortality (bliss of the Wu Wei). It means we are kind with our internal practice and allowed to use the yang energies of impatience, worry, and anger for gathering our fire. All energies are valid: some are just easily misused by being given the wrong goals in which to express their inherent nature.

### *Resolving the Misdirected Energies*

With time and true knowledge, we realign our energies and our earthly desires submit to our heavenly ones. With this achievement, we can transcend the limits of yin and yang and begin to transform them. This transformation does not necessarily progress in a straight line. Like solving a Rubik's cube, we may need to go backward before going forward. Hence, the many variations of hexagrams that life can bestow on us before we can clearly move forward.

As we progress in our practice, we ultimately extract the yang out of Kan and the yin out of Li to produce the hexagram of Tranquillity. This is the fetal state of mind. Then, with further training, we convert each of the yin lines of the Earth trigram (the upper portion of Tranquillity) to yang. This is done by way of Waiting ☷ and Nurturing ☷.

Through this discussion we see that the I Ching is a complex tool that can assist deep understanding of our Kan and Li practice and put much of life into its correct perspective. The sixty-four variations of life circumstances illustrated by the hexagrams are a reflection of the journey of our practice. They teach us that the way our internal energies change is a complex process, which varies despite our superficial will. The hexagrams can also help us realize how the inner is connected to the outer. From this connection a certain letting go and wonderment happens.

## Controlling the Fire and the Steam

Fire and steam, which are fundamental to the process of Kan and Li, need to be properly cultivated and controlled. These adjustments were discussed in detail in *The Practice of Greater Kan and Li* and are summarized below.

In gathering the fire we explore the body with the mind's eye to gather yang energies. We start at a gross level, dissolving tension and unpleasant sensations in our bodies to use these as fire for our coupling. We then work with the natural fires from the heart and adrenals. On occasions fire can rise to the head, and this can be brought down as well. With the progression of training, fire energy becomes more delicate and sophisticated: fine yang energy can be brought down from the stars including spiritual fire from the Three Pure Ones.

To fan the fire—that is, to make it more intense—we suggest several methods. Most of them are ways of increasing your sexual arousal. This can be done through self-stimulation or erotic visualizations, such as a god and goddess making love above you. Changes to the breath can assist this arousal. These breath changes, which include cessation of the breath, making noises with the breath, and bellows breathing, mimic the variety of physiological changes that any couple will go through when having pleasurable intercourse.

Regulating the fire is simply the process of raising and lowering the heat as needed. To reduce the heat, we imagine that the coupling of Kan (tiger) and Li (dragon) occurs in water—a yin environment. To increase the heat, we can couple them in the yang environment of the heavens.

Steaming is the way we obtain purified essence from the organs, channels, and tissues. It is also a way of using a more delicate heating modality for the higher cauldrons of the heart and head. To control the steam, we regulate the fire and make sure there is an adequate supply of water for the cauldron.

## Letting Go

Initially, Kan and Li is hard work with forceful manipulations of the energies in the body so that they couple intensely. This is fine and a great start. As your practice progresses, however, there is more and more letting go and trust in the spontaneous process, allowing for "arresting without arresting and controlling without controlling."[41] With time and practice, one can merely search and center oneself in stillness. With this stillness the coupling will start. It may start very light and small but it soon consumes the whole body and progresses from the lower cauldron to the solar plexus and finally to the heart and head tan tiens. With more delicate and refined efforts, the achievements are less exhausting, more rewarding, and longer lasting.

Just as important as the technique of coupling is the intention behind it. If you have true intention, the coupling and fire regulation will proceed smoothly. True intention takes just as much practice and refinement as the art of coupling itself. Your initial intention may be simply to get the sensation of coupling. Later, you might be motivated by the pleasure of the practice alone. The desire for magical powers may be another reason for doing the practice. Ultimately, however, the practice facilitates the natural coming together of the body's energies. One allows the spirits that dwell in the body to die and merge into the new self—whatever that ends up being. You may feel a sense of self-sacrifice and sadness at the loss of your old self but a little excitement at what the future may bring. In all, there is a gentle trust in the inevitable process.

## Heart as the Site of Coupling

In Greatest Kan and Li practice we move the cauldron to the heart tan tien. This progression in the work includes completing gestation of the spiritual fetus and forming the spiritual infant above the crown. Even when the infant is born, the child can return to the heart position for further nurturing and breast-feeding.

Having the cauldron in the heart serves the following five functions:

1. Education: the cauldron in the heart teaches the fetus how to live in an environment of love and compassion.
2. Merging of the Shen: the Nine Spirits merge into the Higher Shen.
3. Breast-feeding: nurturing the spiritual infant.
4. Opening the chest: helping to remove blockages in the lungs, thymus, and all acupuncture channels that pass through the thorax.
5. Connection with the heart: allows the adept to connect with the pulses of the universe.

### Education

The movement of the coupling to higher and higher levels is a part of the education and development of the fetus. In Lesser Kan and Li, the fetus began knowing its sexual roots. It learned how to be grounded and intimately connected to the earth. The lower cauldron is made of clay and is symbolic of the material nature of Mother Earth. While cooking occurs in all cauldrons, the clay cauldron of the lower tan tien is where a more tangible experience of the earth's healing herbs and plant essences can be cooked and prepared.

The solar plexus cauldron can withstand much higher heat and is made of iron. Now the raw and extreme emotions of the body can be withstood and transformed. The heart is a more delicate cauldron and made of jade. Here, the fetus learns the art of being soft, delicate, and warm. The fetus will understand deeply the transformative powers of love, compassion, and joy.

### Merging of the Shen

In this blissful environment of love, compassion, joy, orgasm, and the presence of the Great Spirit, the Higher Shen chooses to return from the brain to the heart (fig. 3.5). As the chief commander, the Shen

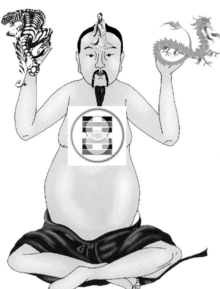

Fig. 3.5. Coupling Kan and Li in the heart to form the Lesser Medicine

can only truly become a leader of the body and its spirits when it sac-rifices itself to a higher good—that of serving the Tao and striving for immortality. The Higher Shen will need to let go of its ego and self-importance and work together with the other spirits as a team of equals. The Great Spirit humbles the Higher Shen into the correct attitude of self-sacrifice. This process of merging of the Shen is known as forming the Lesser Medicine.

### Breast-Feeding

The heart lies between the breasts. In addition to providing sustenance and suckling for the young merged infant, the breasts provide a connec-tion between the heart and the adept's naked sexuality. Suckling is the foundation for many of the UHT practices.

In the womb, where breathing does not occur, suckling is quite active. In high-level meditation external breathing ceases. This is replaced with swallowing of saliva and chi. By regressing the mind and activating this primitive activity, the adept can obtain fetal consciousness. Fetal con-sciousness enables a vision and experience of the Wu Wei.

Suckling forms the foundation experience for kissing and the external practices of Healing Love. In order to have union with the divine, the body has to reactivate this foundational mind-body reflex. Furthermore, suckling also provides a basis for the higher formula of Sealing of the Five Senses. It helps create the ideal position of the lips and facial musculature along with extension of the atlanto-occipital joint.

### Opening the Chest

Many organs and channels run through the chest. Their optimum func-tioning requires good perfusion with chi and blood, which can only be accomplished when the channels are fully open.

Coupling in the heart tan tien facilitates the complete opening of the following channels and organs: the Governing, Conception, Thrusting, Belt, Kidney, Stomach, Spleen, Gall Bladder, Urinary Blad-der, Liver, Lung, Small Intestine, Heart, and Pericardium channels, and the physical structures of the heart, great vessels (aorta and vena cava), lungs, the airways, esophagus, thymus, lymphatics, flesh, and bones of the chest.

### Connection with the Heart

Two basic rhythms form the foundation for our sentient existence: the breath and the heartbeat. It is said that heavenly objects such as the stars also pulsate with life, and many meditative practices that provide access to the unitive state rely on similar foundational rhythms. Our purpose with these formulas is firstly to gain an intimate understanding of the life force behind the heartbeat. Secondly, returning to the heartbeat and breathing that you heard in your mother's womb, and filling your mind with their song, is a way to reaccess fetal consciousness. Further detailed discussion of the importance of the heartbeat will occur in chapter 6.

# Dragon and Tiger

> *The yin tiger shall revert to the position it had before*
> *Khan. And the yang dragon claims its original home at*
> *the center of Li.*
> MIRROR OF THE ALL PERVADING MEDICINE
> OF THE PRIMARY VITALITIES[42]

One of the foundation principles of Kan and Li practice is the mating of the dragon and the tiger.* Such mating involves bringing together two major aspects of consciousness—dimensions of the imagination that form the mythical dragon and the beastly tiger. Both have outward manifestations that are contrary to their inner nature.

---

*The concept of the tiger and the dragon is also used in Fusion meditations, when the practitioner fuses metal with wood. This is also known as the interaction of the green dragon (wood) and the white tiger (metal).

The dragon is a mythical creature that connects to archetypal meanings and images deep in the collective unconscious. It has connections to magic, the dinosaurs of yesteryear, and also to battles of good and evil. Therefore to conjure the power of the dragon you must connect to your dream world. Recall images from your dreams and allow them to permeate the arena of meditation. Understand that the ultimate aim of higher states of mind is the merging of the awakened state, the world of dreams, and the world of meditation. The dragon begins the Kan and Li meditation residing in the house of Li.

Understand the tiger and its nature. It is a beast and a fundamental yet often neglected part of our psyche. It is natural, spontaneous, and both docile and ferocious. Imitate the tiger's nature, yet ground yourself in the quiet space of meditation. The tiger begins Kan and Li meditation residing in the house of Kan.

In Kan and Li practice, the tiger and dragon represent more than just metal and wood. They also have an inner and outer manifestation. They are symbolic of the merging of all phenomena into the duality of Kan and Li. In order to get to this duality we need to use our five-element theory.

The dragon arises from wood and the liver, which originated from the kidneys according to the Creation Cycle or mother-and-son law, but encompasses the element of fire. This means that we need to superimpose those two or three sensations or energies and merge them into one. Though begot from yin (water in the kidneys), the dragon manifests in the house of Li. Its external nature is to fly in the sky and breathe out fire. Its cry is a high-pitched *Eeeeee* sound.[43] Its form consists of stardust (dots of light) and its initial energy is somewhat unpleasant—restless and yang in nature. While the dragon's external manifestation is yang, our experience of it eventually changes to yin. In meditation the dragon causes all things to become moistened. This is its yin component. It is the water in the fire and often cited as the "grease of the dragons."[44]

For the tiger, we may start with feelings in the lungs and a high-frequency metal sensation; we place these into an image of a ferocious feline. The tiger was begotten from fire via the spleen and heart in the creation cycle (mother-son law) or the control cycle (husband-wife law). However, its first appearance manifests in the house of Kan. The tiger is naturally docile and yin, reserving its ferocity and inner fire for the odd occasion. The tiger's roar can be heard as the *Ooommm* sound, and is intimately linked to the sound of the generative force coming from our watery Earth.[45] On initial connection you can sense the tiger's smooth, silk-like fur as well as the cool solid earth that the beast is lying on. However, later—especially when the dragon and tiger interact—you may hear its wild roar and experience the deep pain associated with it. The tiger's inner nature is eventually defined as yang.

The tiger's yang within yin (silver) can be equated to the prenatal essence given from the father's sperm and the mother's blood.* The dragon's yin within yang (grease or mercury) is a condensation of the essence of heaven or the Tao.[46] Many such correspondences between the dragon/tiger and bodily experiences can be identified; the more connections you make, the more powerful the meditation. In particular, connections via the five senses help to awaken experiences of archetypal mythical and magical creatures. For example, the experience of a ringing in the ears awakens awareness of the *Eeeee* sound, which in turn activates the awareness of a high-frequency vibration of the lungs and the stars. The bubbling vibration awakens the dragon from the feet and perineum, which is potentiated by a low frequency *Ooommm* sound seemingly coming from deep within the earth. These sensations act like a portal to deep archetypal connections to the mythical dreamworld. This physical experience of connection is better than simply making an intellectual association with these mythical creatures.

The next stage is to merge or copulate the dragon and the tiger or

---

*The ancient Taoists were not aware of ovulation and believed conception was a result of the fusion of a woman's blood with semen.

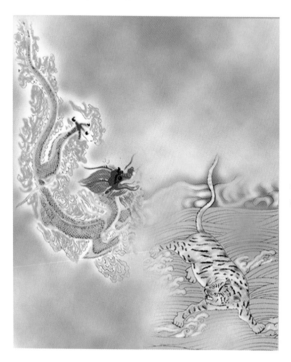

Fig. 3.6. The mating of the dragon and tiger is a form of Kan and Li coupling.

Kan and Li (fig. 3.6). The merging of these two opposites draws out the true yang (mercury) and true yin (silver). Once true yin and yang are identified, they can be finally fused to give rise to an experience of the Golden Elixir of the Tao!

## Merging of the Nine Spirits

> *A human being is a complex individual: immortality implies the unification of spirits and entities that compose and animate the person.*
> SHANQING TAOIST DOCTRINE[47]

The concept of the body and mind containing multiple spirits or personalities has been around for millennia and is a prominent feature of both Eastern and Western thought. In the West, the idea has been discussed at least since the Age of Reason.

William Blake believed that the individual is made up of several spirits. He named these four: Luvah resided in the heart, Urizen (a pun on "you reason") had its home in the head, Tharmas was the spirit of the loins, and Urthona (a pun on "Earth Owner") lay in the earth and cosmos. These deities were endowed with individual powers and abilities, and each one governed certain aspects of the mind and body. Each of these four deities ultimately had to choose between a path of union and one of separate existence.

Separate existence involved diversification, creation of offspring, and disillusionment. The more the individual spirits multiplied, the further they became fragmented and lost. A small remnant of hope and vision remained, however, kindled through the appearance of the immortal Jesus Christ as a bright white light. With the experience of Jesus's pure energy, the four spirits and all their sundry diversifications merge in joyous sexual union. Each spirit had to be prepared to die, however, and sacrifice itself in order to be a part of the One.

This conception of spirit is not too dissimilar from some views held in modern psychology. Carl Jung believed that each person is made up of several archetypes, such as the warrior, the healer, the merchant, etc. The aim of development—which Jung called "individuation"—was the merging of all these archetypes into one integrated being. This is the same goal as the Taoist notion of merging the spirits.

Psychotherapist John Rowan has a notion of salvation that is similar to Blake's: the aim is to discover your inner personalities and get them to work together as a team.[48] Likewise, in the field of psychodrama, the healing occurs when a patient acts out his inner drama, identifying actors who personify the characters within.[49]

The New Age movement offers its version of multiple spirits in the form of past-life regression and spirit guides. The aim of past-life regression therapy is to identify the traumas and attributes of past-life personalities. Once these have been identified, the individual can integrate the positive aspects into her psyche and then let go. Those who are interested in spirit guides first connect with those guides via art, trance work, or the use of an external medium. The next goal is to incorporate these aspects of the hidden self into everyday life.

While all of these therapeutic modalities share certain concepts, each has its own particular medium of expression. Where Jung would use dreams, stories, spontaneous writing, painting, and visions to identify the inner archetypes, psychodrama would use acting to help identify the inner characters. For its part, Taoism uses energy or chi as the key medium. In Taoist Inner Alchemy, spirits have no form but are a particularly refined and integrated kind of energy. Markers of a spirit's origin can be recognized by the senses as color, vibration, and temperature, but they are almost transparent, as spirit energies are even more pure than a child's energy. It often requires the aid of a dark room or cave to discover our spirits; they are self-determined and often experienced as a vortex of chi that is independent of the intellect. Students can use some of the techniques described above to get to know their spirits, even creating an imaginary dialogue to assist in this process.

From a UHT perspective, the inner spirits arise from the heavens and likely originate from a particular star or group of stars, particularly the birth star. The spirits are invoked at the moment of parental orgasm. Conception provides the material housing in which the spirits can develop. In the fetus, the spirits reside in their correct places and work quietly as a team. However, with the process of birth and subsequent growth to adulthood, this harmony is lost, replaced by fragmentation and its ensuing consequences.

The Taoist Inner Alchemy system does offer a way home, however. Fabrizio Pregadio summarizes the classical understanding of the spirits below:

> They act as offices in the bureaucratic system that manages the whole body; they perform healing tasks by supporting the balance of the body's functions; and they are objects of meditation. The basic purpose of visualizing them is to "maintain" them in their proper loca-

tions, nourish them with one's inner breaths and essences, and invoke them so that in turn they provide protection and sustenance. This is said to ensure health, longevity, or immortality, and to defend one from calamities caused by demons and other noxious entities.[50]

Firstly, each of the spirits belongs to a bureaucratic system and has its correct location. For example, the Shen in the heart, merged with the Higher Shen, is the supreme commander. The other organ spirits serve the Shen: the kidney spirit is responsible for willpower, while the Yi of the spleen governs thinking. The Hun forms the dream body, and the Po is concerned more with immediate and materialistic desires.

Unfortunately, what happens as we "grow up" is that the spirits become fragmented: each can become self important and self-serving. For example, the Yi—the thinking component of the spleen (horse intellect)—can deny the emotional aspects of the solid organs. It can indulge itself in excessive mind chatter and intellectual problem solving. One then becomes too monkey minded with suppressed emotions and consequent imbalance. Sexuality, the Zhi spirit of the kidneys, can take over the mind and try to drive the whole person toward destructive sexuality. The Higher Shen can take over as a militant leader and suppress all other spirits because it has no faith in their separate abilities.

There is variation among the various Taoist sects as to the exact number and location of the spirits. In the UHT system, there are nine spirits altogether. In Ge Hong's time, Hussein cites three spirits and seven souls.[51] In the Shanqing era they meditated on the nine spirits in the head alone that occupied the Nine Palaces of the brain.[52] In Lingbao Taoism the body contained twenty-four deities.[53] In all cases, health and immortality involves each of the spirits returning to its ideal functioning and operating from its own space. These are outlined in the table on page 84.

The student is probably aware of the five organ spirits. In the UHT system there is also one above the head that is yin and another inside the

head that is yang. There is a spirit behind the knees and a soul beneath
the feet, totalling nine. The difference between a soul and a spirit is a
small point, and lengthy discussion of it is beyond the confines of this
text. In brief, however, a soul is more heavy, inward, and quiet. It is yin
and hence can be used with Kan in the coupling process. It may have
a memory of its former existence and goes to the earth after death.
The spirit is more outward and comes from the light of the heavens.
It is yang, outward, louder, and perhaps unpleasant at times. It can be
located initially in the house of Li.

## LOCATION AND FUNCTION OF THE NINE SPIRITS

| LOCATION | SPIRIT/SOUL NAME | FUNCTION |
| --- | --- | --- |
| **Above crown** | Highest Soul | Serves to connect to heaven |
| **Brain** | Higher Shen (spirit) | Combines with shen to form Yi (Heart-mind power/Supreme Commander) |
| **Heart** | Shen (spirit) | Enthusiasm |
| **Spleen** | Yi (spirit) | Problem solving |
| **Lung** | Po (soul) | Corporeal soul (manifestation) |
| **Kidney** | Zhi (spirit) | Willpower |
| **Liver** | Hun (soul) | Ethereal soul—connected to dream body, planning and vision |
| **Behind knees** | (spirit) | Spare spirit (back-up for others) |
| **Below feet** | Unknown Chinese name (soul) | Serves to connect to the earth |

The activity of visualizing the spirits and meditating on them is a
process of invocation. Each spirit is invoked when it is uniquely identified through direct experience in meditation using all of the senses along
with imaginary dialogue. Dreams and other life interests can also help to
identify the spirits as outlined in the above discussion of modern therapeutic modalities. This is how each spirit is nourished and how "breath"
and essence are given to each of them. Through this process, the needs,

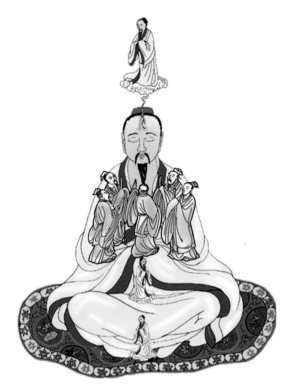

Fig. 3.7. Location of the Nine Spirits within the body

wants, and issues of the spirits can be met and the process of unification begins. With this healing, we can begin to collect our energies into a team, viewing even our demons as our own energies working toward the wrong goal. If we can manage to get all our spirits and souls to work together, then the demons and noxious entities will be exorcized. This reframing will reverse destructive tendencies, allowing them to provide sustenance and protection instead.

Ultimately, each spirit is educated to the point of understanding the importance of serving the higher good through self-sacrifice to the whole. This humbling step is enabled by direct meditative experience of the Great Spirit (Taiyi) as overwhelming light. Kan and Li practice furthers the greater good by helping each spirit revert to its original purpose and position. In Lesser Kan and Li practice, the liver soul seeds the cauldron and fuses with the embryo in the lower tan tien. In Greater Kan and Li the Spleen spirit fuses with the fetus in the solar plexus. Finally, in

Greatest Kan and Li, the Higher Shen leaves the head to merge with the fetus in the heart. Eventually all must combine to find new meaning with virtue and compassion. The whole then can become the Original Spirit (Yuan Shen) reborn through the spiritual embryo.

Once the embryo completes its gestation it can be reborn and raised into the spiritual body. Once a spiritual body is raised the spirits can return home to its star and be absorbed into the Wu Wei.

## Pole Stars and Associated Constellations

The Pole Star Polaris is less than one degree from the North Celestial Pole. It is the brightest star of the constellation of Ursa Minor, with a magnitude near 2. (Note that the lower the magnitude the brighter the star.) Mars and Saturn are just a little brighter than Polaris.

The North Pole Star and the Big Dipper have played a crucial role in Taoist practice since shamanic times, when the legendary Wu performed a ritual spiral dance marking a journey from the outer multitude of stars to the Big Dipper and finally to the Pole Star.

The early Taoists could see the constellations spiralling inwardly toward the Pole Star, and they understood that dynamic to be a mirror of our earthly existence and our minds (fig. 3.8). In this view, our journey from fragmentation and disillusionment is a slow inward spiral toward salvation and peace. The multitude of constellations represents the many facets of everyday existence. But as we experience these from the ground up and learn the appropriate lessons, we let go and move closer to the still center. The task was to marry our awake world, our dream (spirit) world, and our meditation world in accordance with the play of stars in the firmament.

From a meditation perspective, the Pole Star is a gate to the stillness of the Wu Wei. We have a multitude of energies, sensations, and thoughts: with practice we can condense these energies into the one energy of the

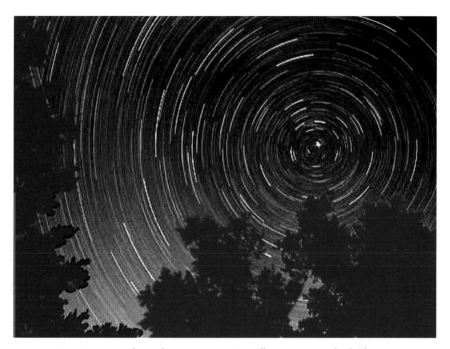

Fig. 3.8. The Pole Star acts as a still point around which
the multiple constellations revolve.

primordial—a process that matches the journey of the stars condensing
into one point at the Pole Star. We start by connecting the Pole Star to the
Ba Hui and Crystal Palace. Later, in Greater Kan and Li practice, we begin
to learn vertical flight to this place. Once we find our heart truly opening
in the Greatest Kan and Li, we can align our own heart with the heart of
heaven so that they are one. We project our bodies across the entire visible
universe on a path paved by the twenty-eight Lunar Mansions. It is from
this state of mind that we can find our rest as a heavenly being.

In the world of dreams and spirits, the Pole Star connects us to the
Three Pure Ones, who have the ability to dissolve the Three Worms.[54]
The Pole Star represents unification and solidarity; it is through this
mechanism that it gains its secret apotrophatic (exorcizing) powers.

In the material world, the Pole Star represents the center and foundation through which all disparate energies can find a common goal. This

is, of course, love and compassion through our heart center. The Pole Star can thus be regarded as the heart of heaven,[55] as seen in the Chart of the Inner Warp (Neijing Tu) (fig. 3.9).[56] As far as the earth is concerned, the Pole Star represents Mount Kun Lun. Like the heart, this mountain is the focal point around which the earth meridians and energy lines need to meet for ideal harmony.

When we connect with the heart of heaven, we encounter a deeply healing violet chi, which triggers a cascade of regeneration that counters our usual aging and degeneration processes.

### Big Dipper

The Big Dipper is part of the constellation of Ursa Major. Its seven stars are named Dubhe, Merak, Phecda, Megrez, Elioth, Miza, and Alkaid. The magnitude of these stars varies from 1.8 to 3.3.

### STARS OF THE BIG DIPPER, WITH CRANIAL BONE AND BRAIN CORRESPONDENCES

| STAR | CHINESE NAME | CRANIAL BONE | BRAIN |
|------|--------------|--------------|-------|
| 1. α Dubhe | Hungry Wolf/ Bright Yang | Left Mastoid | Cerebellum |
| 2. β Merak | Huge Gate/Yin Essence | Right Mastoid | Memory Center |
| 3. γ Phecda | Pure Person/ Prosperity Storage | Right Temple/ Cheekbone | Pineal Gland |
| 4. δ Megrez | Intellectual Art/ Mystic Subtlety | Left Temple/ Cheekbone | |
| 5. ε Elioth | Honest Chastity/ Prime Elixir | Chin | Thalamus |
| 6. ζ Miza | Martial Art/North Pole | Base of Skull | |
| 7. η Alkaid | Destructive Army/ Heavenly Guard | Anterior Fontanelle (Coronal and Sagittal Suture) | |

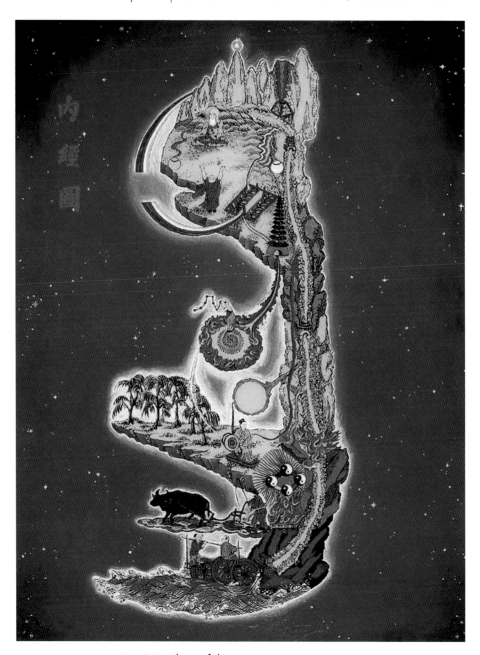

Fig. 3.9. Chart of the Inner Warp (Neijing Tu),
showing the Pole Star as the heart center with an inward spiral
and the Big Dipper surrounding it

Like the Pole Star, the Big Dipper holds a notable position among the stellar objects as a vital step toward immortality. It gains its role through both its shape and proximity to the Pole Star, which can be found by allocating five lengths of the cup between Dubhe and Merak.

The Big Dipper's shape is that of a ladle with a long handle and deep bowl. The bowl is for gathering pure essence from the North Star and pouring this down upon the meditator in the manner of a baptism. The Dipper thus acts as a vehicle for delivering the pure essence of the Three Pure Ones. This pure essence is the antidote to the forces of the Three Death Bringers (Three Worms).

The ladle is made up of seven stars, although some Taoist schools quote nine. There are apparently two hidden stars, Fu and Bi, which only advanced adepts can see.[57] They are located on either side of Alkaid. These extra two stars then allow the Dipper to represent the Nine Palaces, Nine Orifices, Nine Mountains, and the Nine Spirits.

The other function of the Big Dipper is to act as a key that enables access to the Pole Star and ultimately to visions of the Wu Wei. This can be done in several ways. The first way is to separate the cranial bones and consequently open the suture lines and acupuncture channels that cross the skull. The other formula, which is included in *The Taoist Soul Body*,* allows practitioners to connect the stars of the Big Dipper to vital parts of the brain, including the cerebellum, memory center, pineal gland, thalamus, hypothalamus, pituitary gland, and third eye. The secret here is to turn off the cerebral cortex—with its associated monkey mind—and tune in to the more primitive parts of the brain associated with naturalness and spontaneity. The monkey mind then tranforms into the meditative mystical mind, which is intimately connected to third-eye experiences.

Some Taoist sects advocate reversing the handle of the Big Dipper in order to reverse aging.[58] Since the handle points outward toward the myriad of stars and multiplicity, and the tip of the cup is closest to the

---

*Additional formulas and explanations of the Big Dipper can be found in the Lesser Kan and Li text, *The Taoist Soul Body* (Rochester, Vt.: Destiny Books, 2007).

Pole Star and hence the most centered aspect of the Big Dipper, then reducing multiplicity is in essence the reversing of the handle, thereby bringing it closer to the Pole Star.

### Southern Cross and the South Celestial Pole

Now that the Taoist practices are becoming worldwide, suggestions are being made about appropriate constellations for southern practitioners. While there is no information about southern stars available in either Taoist or other Internal Alchemical traditions, it is noted that the Australian aboriginals cite the importance of the Southern Cross. They described it as a stingray with its tail pointing toward the South Celestial Pole (fig. 3.10). The two pointers, Alpha and Beta Centauri, are described as sharks or as two legendary brothers who escaped a fire by flying and then took up residence in the sky. Most aboriginal tribes believed that animals and humans would reside in the sky as immortals (in the dreamtime) following heroic deeds.

The South Celestial Pole is marked by Sigma Octantis (Polaris Australis). It has a magnitude of 5.45 and is hence not visible in urban

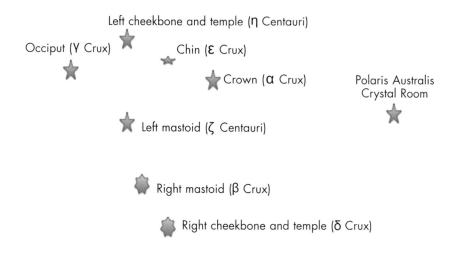

Fig. 3.10. South Celestial Pole, Southern Cross,
Alpha and Beta Centauri

environments; it can barely be seen with the naked eye even under ideal conditions. However, a good set of binoculars will ensure its sighting. It is one degree from the South Celestial Pole.

The Southern Cross (the Crux constellation) and its two pointers, Alpha and Beta Centauri (part of the Centaurus constellation), together comprise seven stars. Like its counterpart the Big Dipper, the Southern Cross appears on national flags. The axis of the Crux points toward the South Celestial Pole, which is approximately 4.5 lengths of the Crux. The Pole can also be found by drawing a perpendicular axis through the two pointers, Alpha and Beta Centauri.

Some practitioners recommend using only the five stars of the Crux for the southern meditations.[59] However, this approach denies the correspondences set up for a seven-star system. A seven-star model would include the correspondences cited in the table and fig. 3.10 on the previous page. Associated stars of lower magnitude such as Zeta and Yeta Crux would make up the nine.

## SEVEN-STAR CORRESPONDENCES
## TO CRANIAL BONES, SOUTHERN SKY

| STAR | CRANIAL BONE | BRAIN |
|---|---|---|
| 1. α Crux | Anterior Fontanelle | Third Eye |
| 2. β Crux | Right Mastoid | Pineal Gland |
| 3. γ Crux | Base of Occiput | Cerebellum |
| 4. δ Crux | Right Cheekbone | Memory Center |
| 5. ε Crux | Chin | Olfactory Gland/Pituitary |
| 6. ζ Centauri | Left Mastoid | Hypothalamus |
| 7. η Centauri | Left Cheekbone | Thalamus |

# Heavenly Stems and Earthly Branches (Ganzhi) and the Twenty-Eight Lunar Mansions

The Heavenly Stems and Earthly Branches represent an ordinal method of dissecting the infinite realm of time and space into smaller defined pieces. Note that the ten stems reside in their celestial origins, while their influence branches into the earth. This system began as an ancient calendar. Geomancers use it to predict inauspicious and auspicious times, while Taoist Inner Alchemy adepts use it for condensing time and space to discover the "one."

This method of subdivision, which uses a sexagesimal system, began in the Shang era (approximately 1500 BCE). However, a sexagesimal system appeared in Mesopotamia around 3000 BCE, therefore the Chinese system may have originated there.* Shang-era astronomers divided time into twelve-year cycles (based on the twelve-year orbit of Jupiter) and ten-day weeks (based on the five elements with subdivisions of yin and yang). The ten Heavenly Stems named the different days of the week. Each day was unique, reflected by the stem that produced a new sun for that day. The twelve Earthly Branches, based on the Chinese zodiacal animals, named each of twelve two-hour periods of the twenty-four-hour day. A unique combination of the ten-day week and half of the Heavenly Stems produced a sixty-day year ($0.5 \times 10 \times 12$).

The days of these cycles were connected to the twenty-eight Lunar Mansions (constellations) that the moon traverses in its twenty-eight-day cycle around the ecliptic. The choice of the number twenty-eight may also be derived from the number of years it takes for Saturn to orbit the Sun.† The lunar mansions do not fit exactly into the stems and branches calendar system. The moon takes twenty-nine to thirty days to complete the cycle from new moon to new moon. So it takes less than three ten-day

---

*Despite this calendar being confusing to the modern reader, the sexagesimal system is a wonderful system, as there are 360 degrees in a circle and it is divisible by more numbers than a decimal system.

†The actual average is 29.5 years for Saturn's year.

weeks to complete its journey around the earth. The lunar calendar year is about eleven days short of the 365-day solar year. These are caught up in leap years when an extra month is added to the calendar. (Note that these leap years don't coincide with the leap years of the Gregorian calendar.) The new sexagesimal year starts in the Northern Hemisphere with the second new moon after the winter solstice (as long as this moon does not appear before January 21). If the second new moon does appear before January 21, an extra month is added to the calendar.

The twenty-eight-day cycle is divided into four quarters that correspond to the four directions and standard totem animals (also see fig. 3.11 on page 97): north is the Turtle, east the Green Dragon, west the White Tiger, south the Red Pheasant, while the Yellow Phoenix occupies the central earth position. Each quadrant is divided into seven constellations or Lunar Mansions.

## THE TWENTY-EIGHT LUNAR MANSIONS AND ASSOCIATED WESTERN CONSTELLATIONS

| TOTEM ANIMAL | NO. | CHINESE NAME | TRANSLATION | CONSTELLATION |
|---|---|---|---|---|
| Green dragon | 1 | Jiao | Horn | Virgo |
| | 2 | Kang | Neck | Virgo |
| | 3 | Di | Root | Scorpio |
| | 4 | Fung | Room | Scorpio |
| | 5 | Hsing | Heart | Scorpio |
| | 6 | Wey | Tail | Scorpio |
| | 7 | Ji | Basket | Sagitarrius |
| Black tortoise | 8 | Do | Dipper (South) | Sagitarrius |
| | 9 | Niu | Ox | Capricorn |
| | 10 | Nu | Female | Aquarius |
| | 11 | Xu | Emptiness | Aquarius |
| | 12 | Wey | Roof | Aquarius |

| TOTEM ANIMAL | NO. | CHINESE NAME | TRANSLATION | CONSTELLATION |
|---|---|---|---|---|
| | 13 | Shi | Encampment | Pegasus (adjacent to Pisces) |
| | 14 | Bie | Wall | Pegasus (adjacent to Pisces) |
| White tiger | 15 | Kui | Legs | Andromeda (adjacent to Pisces) |
| | 16 | Lou | Bond | Aries |
| | 17 | Wei | Stomach | Aries |
| | 18 | Mao | Head | Taurus |
| | 19 | Bi | Net | Taurus |
| | 20 | Zi | Turtle Mouth | Orion (adjacent to Taurus) |
| | 21 | Shen | Three Stars | Orion (adjacent to Gemini) |
| Red pheasant | 22 | Qing | Well | Gemini |
| | 23 | Quei | Ghost | Cancer |
| | 24 | Liu | Willow | Hydra (adjacent to Leo) |
| | 25 | Hsing | Star | Hydra (adjacent to Leo) |
| | 26 | Chang | Large Net | Hydra (adjacent to Leo) |
| | 27 | Yi | Wings | Crater (adjacent to Virgo) |
| | 28 | Chen | Chariot | Corvus (adjacent to Virgo) |

In this system, a solar year initially consisted of 360 days, each of which was divided into two-hour sectors, for a total of twelve time periods. These time periods again correspond to the twelve animals of the zodiac. Geographically, the twelve time periods divided the earth into thirty-degree arcs. Given the earth's rotation over a twenty-four hour period, the Earthly Branches numbering twelve can cover the entire planet (see fig. 3.12 on page 97).

Thus the Heavenly Stems and Earthly Branches connect time to the planets and their orbits, to the constellations and stars through the Lunar Mansions, and in turn to all phenomena through interplay of the elements with the animal zodiac. Time (the ten Heavenly Stems via the five visible planets and yin and yang) takes on a new meaning, based on the geography and constituents of the universe. The rotation and orbits of the heavenly bodies manifest the forces of Heavenly Chi.

### HEAVENLY STEMS WITH THEIR PLANETARY AND ELEMENTAL CORRESPONDENCES

| | CHINESE CHARACTER | HEAVENLY STEM | YIN YANG | ELEMENT | PLANET |
|---|---|---|---|---|---|
| 1 | 甲 | Jia | Yang | Wood | Jupiter |
| 2 | 乙 | Yi | Yin | | |
| 3 | 丙 | Bing | Yang | Fire | Mars |
| 4 | 丁 | Ding | Yin | | |
| 5 | 戊 | Wu | Yang | Earth | Saturn |
| 6 | 己 | Ji | Yin | | |
| 7 | 庚 | Geng | Yang | Metal | Venus |
| 8 | 辛 | Xin | Yin | | |
| 9 | 壬 | Ren | Yang | Water | Mercury |
| 10 | 癸 | Gui | Yin | | |

### The Power of Connecting to the Heavenly Stems and Earthly Branches

For the meditator, connecting to the Heavenly Stems means connecting with time and space via the planetary and stellar bodies and their inherent rotations and orbits. To do this, the meditator methodically connects to the visible planets and the constellations one by one. Because the Lunar Mansions are so many and unfamiliar, it is our opinion that substitution

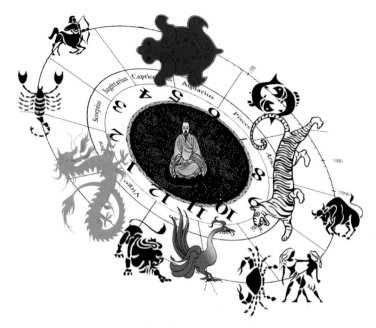

Fig. 3.11. Four mythical creatures and their quadrants:
the Lunar Mansions and the Western zodiac

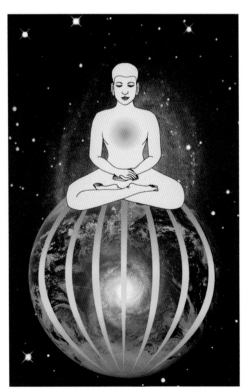

Fig. 3.12. Meditator dividing
the earth with twelve thirty-
degree arcs, creating twelve
two-hour time periods

of the Western zodiac provides a useful compromise. The Lunar Mansions and Western zodiac have much crossover and the table below highlights this. The non-zodiac constellations of Hydrae, Pegasus, and Andromeda are included. These also border the ecliptic.

The adept can learn the Western constellations by rote and thus generate a genuine meditative connection with the stars. This diligent though vast connection assists the mind in connecting with heavenly force and ultimately in condensing the heavens into one sensation.

## TWELVE EARTHLY BRANCHES WITH THEIR ANIMAL AND TIME-PERIOD CORRESPONDENCES

|  | EARTHLY BRANCH | CHINESE | ANIMAL | TWO-HOUR PERIOD |
|---|---|---|---|---|
| 1 | 子 | Zi | Rat | 11 p.m.–1 a.m. |
| 2 | 丑 | Chou | Buffalo | 1–3 a.m. |
| 3 | 寅 | Yin | Tiger | 3–5 a.m. |
| 4 | 卯 | Mao | Rabbit | 5–7 a.m. |
| 5 | 辰 | Chen | Dragon | 7–9 a.m. |
| 6 | 巳 | Si | Snake | 9–11 a.m. |
| 7 | 午 | Wu | Horse | 11 a.m.–1 p.m. |
| 8 | 未 | Wei | Goat | 1–3 p.m. |
| 9 | 申 | Shen | Monkey | 3–5 p.m. |
| 10 | 酉 | You | Rooster | 5–7 p.m. |
| 11 | 戌 | Xu | Dog | 7–9 p.m. |
| 12 | 亥 | Hai | Pig | 9–11 p.m. |

Likewise, connecting to the Earthly Branches enables access to earthly time, geography, and the life force of living and inanimate creatures. In a stepwise fashion, the meditator can throw pearls around the earth at thirty-degree intervals. Once the entire globe is covered and a sensation of connecting to everything in it is complete, the adept can summate the earth's force as one energetic sensation.

## RESOLVING THE FINAL DUALITIES

### Heaven and Earth (Space), Past and Future (Time), the Observer and the Observed

*Tao is mind, mind is the mind of the Tao, body is the body of Tao, sharing the qualities of heaven and earth, sharing the light of the sun and the moon, sharing the order of the seasons—the whole world is within one's body.*

LIU I-MING[60]

In the Greatest Kan and Li practice, our purpose is to merge the triad of time, space, and observership. In alchemy, not one stone, not one living creature, not one aliquot of time is neglected. In order to reach the One, the whole must be embraced. We condense all the animating forces into a duality of Heaven and Earth. Through the power of Kan and Li practice, Earth submits to Heaven and is subsumed into nothingness.

## Heaven and Earth: Space

In the Lesser Kan and Li meditation we worked with grosser and perhaps more contaminated energies of Kan and Li. Our purpose was really to cleanse and purify the body. In order to realize the One, the body must be first embraced. To forget oneself to a greater whole, the adept must include every square millimeter of the bodily self. The Lesser Kan and Li meditation accomplishes this by steaming the organs and connecting to all the acupuncture channels. It specifically focuses on the Bridge and Regulator channels.

The Greater Kan and Li meditations teach the adept to begin geographical expansion beyond the self. This is initially taught in the Greater Kan and Li warm-ups via the Unicorn Practice, Vertical Flight, and Earth Flight practices. These meditations extend the adept's awareness beyond the confines of the body to parts of the earthly realm (including the underworld) and then to the perimeter of the solar system.

The mind can leave the confines of the physical body via the third eye, the crown, or the root chakra. Through these portals the adept can experience a deep sense of outer space. In this way, the adept explores the solar system and the specific nature of the planets, sun, and moon. Like the Greek and Roman cultures, the ancient Chinese regarded the visible planets as the realm of the immortals. To become an immortal one must digest, absorb, and sexually unite with these planetary deities. At times, the adept will imagine a particular planet and then feel a surge of energy. In some respects, it is as if the adept digests or absorbs the energy of that planet. Perhaps at this instant, the adept takes on the planet's godlike or immortal qualities.

Beyond the solar system lie other solar systems, constellations, and galaxies. To embrace the One the adept must connect with the entirety of the universe. This connection takes place over time, as the adept progresses through the Kan and Li series and Sealing of the Five Senses meditations. This spatial expansion of self is one of the three basic requirements for the realization of the unitive experience.

## Past and Future: Time

The compression of time into the moment is not taught overtly by the formulas like the geographical expansion. However, time and geography are intimately connected. With the Heavenly Stems and Earthly Branches we connect to time through the spinning of the earth and the orbits of the planetary and stellar bodies. Likewise in astral travel, time can be altered via entry into wormholes, wherein the mind travels faster than the speed of light.

Like each part of the body and the universe, the past must be embraced. It is only then that one can let go of it. Not embracing the past creates an unconscious agenda that takes us away from our ultimate purpose. Remember the original spirit yearns only to join the entire history of the universe. This means that every positive historical event is directing you toward this goal. Every negative historical event is also contextualized in this framework. Any other interpretation of your personal history or the earth's history is counterproductive. Therefore feel every measure of time gathering momentum toward your ultimate quest. Likewise, let go of the future. The future has an aura of expectation. This is the dark side of the formulas that we teach you. Expect too much and the future exists. Have no expectation and the future dies into the moment.

Eventually with successful meditation, the adept trusts and lets go. All dissolves into the pleasure of the now. The now is infinite and includes the past and the future if you will allow it. Time is in the moment and all the aeons are compressed. The adept begins to understand spatial unity and now the infinite time of the moment. These two aspects ebb and flow into each other but are not complete until the self is destroyed.

## Observer and the Observed:
## Death of the Observer

> *Not a single thought arises; he who is looking inward*
> *suddenly forgets that he is looking.*
>
> Lu Dong-Pin[61]

The journey to death of self is a long one. It begins with the adept discovering each of his fragmented parts, via the aid of the five-element theory and the pakua theory of the eight forces. By learning, identifying, and owning the various correspondences, the adept begins to complete a picture of himself. In the Greater Kan and Li practice, these parts of self are realized through energetic connection to body parts, virgin children, animals, and plants. Everything in the phenomenal world is symbolic of parts of our self. Unfortunately, beyond the joy of discovery of a forgotten part of us comes the realization that this part must soon die. This death occurs through the power of sexual desire, when we merge all of our small parts into one whole (fig. 3.13).

Inherent in the Kan and Li formulas is the principle that when two opposites are coupled, something new is born. Sexual energy is the vehicle for creating something new out of disparate parts. From another perspective, this something new is also a miniature death. This small death is the death of our old fragmented self and birth to the larger whole.

Eventually, this whole grows to encompass the marriage of Heaven and Earth. In meditation our sense of self is identified by tension in the body and thoughts that arise. "I exist and am separate because I have tension in my body!" Alternatively, we have Descartes' opinion, "I think, therefore I exist." In meditation practice, this thinking is intimately linked with the mind-state of observing. It involves observing the identification and interpretation of conscious awareness.

As one drifts into stillness, the sense of self begins to fall apart. Like Chuang-tzu in his famous eulogy that praises loss of self-awareness with a butterfly, we find our minds asking a similar question: "Is the universe watching me or is it me watching the universe?" The ultimate union of self and the universe—the congress of heaven and man—occurs when this question is answered. The answer cannot be answered in words but surely lies in the realm of forgetting!

When the triad is complete, a new reality is forged. The ultimate

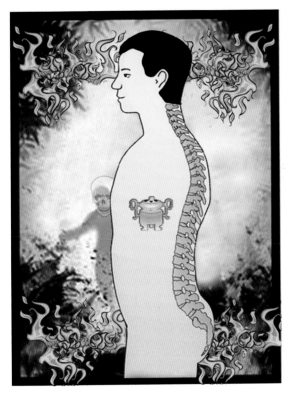

Fig. 3.13. Death of the observer as
he is born again into the Whole

death and rebirth takes the adept into a mystery. This mystery can be
called immortality and is easily achieved by any devoted student. You
don't need to belong to a church and you don't require a miracle. All you
need to do is practice! We hope the reader understands these concepts
and makes them a reality.

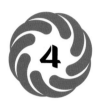

# Warm-Ups for Self-Practice

This chapter includes six techniques that are appropriate to use as warm-ups prior to entering the Kan and Li phase of your sitting meditation. These warm-ups include Sexual Practices, Elixir Chi Kung, Pulsing, Merging the Dragon and the Tiger, Invocation of the Three Pure Ones, and Expelling the Three Worms. Note that in *The Practice of Greater Kan and Li* we offered other warm-up practices, including the Inner Smile, Fusion, Embryonic Respiration, and Spiraling (Unicorn, Vertical, and Earth flight). The student can choose to use any or a combination of these methods to prepare for formal Kan and Li Practice.

## SEXUAL PRACTICES

Without sexual desire the meditations of Kan and Li become difficult if not impossible. The whole concept of Kan and Li relies on the control of sexual energy. Therefore the male sexual practices of Semen Retention, Testicular Breathing, Scrotal Compression, Power Lock, Chi Weight Lifting, and Orgasmic Upward Draw are vital to the success of advanced Inner Alchemy practice. For women, the reduction of menses, Ovarian Breathing, Vaginal Compression,

Orgasmic Upward Draw, and Egg Techniques are vital for successful Kan and Li practice.

When sexual practices are used as a warm-up, they can be done via solo or dual cultivation. In solo practice, the purpose is to both create and use sexual energy (Ching Chi) to awaken the orgasm energy, which in turn can be used to open the various channels of the body. The orgasm energy is ultimately a vibrating self-contained chi ball that can be moved wherever it needs to go to open up blocked areas of the body. The Orgasmic Upward Draw, for example, moves the orgasm energy up the spine along the Governing Channel to awaken key Governing Vessel points (fig. 4.1). Remember that by opening up the spine at these key points there will be automatic improvement in chi flow to the various solid and hollow organs.

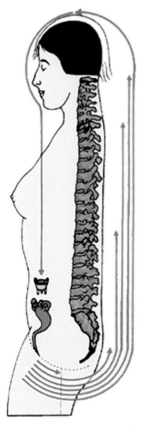

Fig. 4.1. The Orgasmic Upward Draw can be used as a warm-up exercise for Kan and Li practice.

As you direct the vibrating Ching Chi or orgasm energy, you can feel the organ soften and chi flowing to that organ. Finally, the Orgasm Chi is taken to the brain with involution of the senses. The practice can end with bringing the combined chi down the Conception Vessel.

When using sexual energy, you may find that your sexual desire is associated with past lovemaking experiences or fantasy scenes. Do not be judgmental of these and also don't overuse them in your practice. Remember that while your mind is in a memory or fantasy image, your energy is not entirely with you. Part of your mind is in the future or past, and thus it is not totally focussed on the present. For some novices, sexual fantasies are the only way that they can get started and feel anything. With time, they can gently allow these people-images to disappear. This is called purification of Ching Chi.

If possible, gently allow the orgasm to be replaced by the interplay between the energies of Kan and Li in the lower tan tien. This is a natural transition between the Orgasmic Upward Draw and the coupling of Kan and Li. Once coupling has occurred in the lower tan tien for a while and the organs have been steamed, you can move the coupling to the solar plexus and then to the heart.

# ELIXIR CHI KUNG
# (SWALLOWING SALIVA)

Saliva is renowned as the water of life. Swallowing saliva is part of the pathway to immortality. However, it belongs to the whole complex of changes that mark the shift from adult to embryonic existence. When one has a deep meditation experience such as expansion of consciousness via vertical, horizontal, or subterranean flight, or in the coupling of Kan and Li, respiration stops and the swallowing reflex kicks in.*

The exact nature of this reflex can be explained as regression to embry-

---

*See chapter 7 for a more detailed discussion of saliva practice.

onic physiology. When you were an embryo—and there was no air to breathe—you benefited from primitive reflexes that helped to improve your circulation. The swallowing reflex could help the body relax and open its channels.

When the adept is coupling deeply, lots of other physical responses also arise, including the empty force breath against a closed glottis and moments of packing the breath. There is a move away from the fragmented material world to the energetic realm of immortality wherein a whole lot of embryonic and primitive reflexes kick in. Universal Healing Tao training tries to teach you these consciously so that when they occur naturally they are nurtured and prioritized. Remember the whole of the Kan and Li practice is a return to what is natural and a return to the embryonic state of being. From there the state of immortality can be achieved.

 ## Swallowing Saliva Warm-Up Practice

1. Begin with the Inner Smile practice.
2. With your mouth lightly closed, be aware of the mouth, the nose, and the eyes. Inhale very slowly and lightly press the tip of the tongue to the palate, feeling that you are drawing in the smiling energy—the essence of the air—into the eyes, nose, and mouth. When you exhale, condense this essence in the mouth. Do this 9 to 18 times until you feel that the tongue and the palate have a connection.
3. Feel electric vibrations in the tongue, palate, saliva glands, and the glands of the brain. This is the natural way of stimulating and strengthening these glands. Be aware of and picture the pituitary gland and feel the vibration reaching it. Be aware of and picture the hypothalamus and pineal glands and feel the electric vibration stimulating these glands.
4. Feel the saliva starting to flow even more and the vibration going deeper and deeper into the brain. The palate is very porous and

hormonal secretions start to drip down from the roof of the mouth. These secretions taste different from saliva—thicker, sweeter, and more fragrant. Use the tongue to sweep around and gather the nectar.

5. When you've gathered a mouthful of saliva, move your tongue around like you are chewing and eating delicious food, mixing it well. Move the saliva back and forth, left and right, up and down, to mix it with all the essences, hormones, and the air.

6. As you deepen in your meditation, absorb the forces that you sense around you, such as bubbling water, fire, thunder, lake (still water), earth, mountain, wind, and heaven, and allow the swallowing reflex to begin (fig. 4.2). Very slightly prevent yourself from breathing—just enough to encourage the swallowing process.

7. Continue with a deepening of the meditation and allow the forces to take over the body and mind. With this deepening, allow the breath

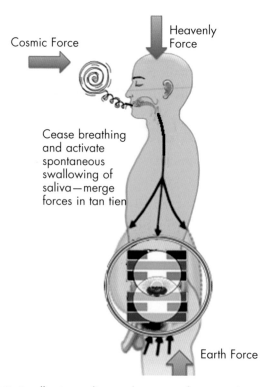

Fig. 4.2. Swallowing saliva and merging forces in the tan tien

to almost cease as you continue to swallow saliva while absorbing and merging the various forces.

8. At this stage you may enter into the formal coupling of Kan and Li.

# PULSING

Pulsing is the body's way of maintaining energetic homeostasis (balance) of the body. From an experiential perspective in meditation, concentrating the mind on pulsing dissolves blockages and opens channels. Thus pulsing improves and advances the meditation experience. In the *Yellow Emperor's Classic of Internal Medicine* (Huangdi Neijing Suwen), pulsing is recommended for "the development and perfection of the five orbs." It says, "red also corresponds to the pulse . . . the pulse is connected to the eyes."[1] Ishida tells us that, "The pulse is another form of energy closely related to the protective and constructive energies, as well as to great primordial energy of life itself. One can imagine pulse as waves of the various fluids flying around the body."[2]

 ## Pulsing Practice

In the Lesser Kan and Li practice, pulsing is used as a formal meditation, introduced after coupling; here in the Greatest Kan and Li practice it is suggested as a warm-up.

1. Allow the body to relax, then begin by feeling one pulse in your body. A good pulse to start with is one within the head. However, any pulse that comes to attention is worthwhile.
2. Mentally allow the heart rate to decrease.
3. Amplify the strength of the pulse at the crown and perineum points. This will assist the heart by moving the blood with chi energy.
4. Amplify the pulse at the navel, groin, inner ankles, and feet.
5. Amplify the pulse at the neck, temple, back of skull, armpits, inside elbows, and wrists.

6. As you become familiar with this exercise, begin to synchronize all pulses (fig. 4.3). By re-creating the pulse in other areas, you will eventually be able to transfer the pulse to the lower tan tien and use this to facilitate coupling. Pulsing harmonizes with the coupling and accentuates it.

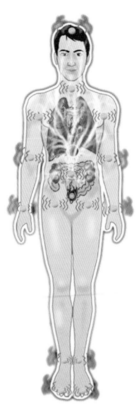

Fig. 4.3. Pulsing practice

Pulsing can be combined with other rhythms like spiraling and is potentially a vehicle for mystical experience in its own right.

## MERGING THE DRAGON AND TIGER

As discussed in chapter 3, the mating of the dragon and tiger is intimately related to the coupling of Kan and Li.

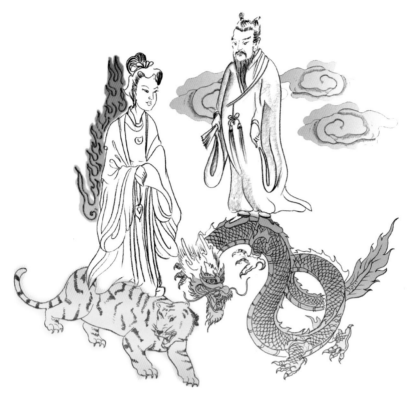

Fig. 4.4. Dragon and tiger playing and
mating as a warm-up meditation

## Merging the Dragon and Tiger

1. Identify the dragon and tiger in your imagination; then let them play according to their volition (fig. 4.4).
2. Hear the sounds of the dragon (*Eeeeee* sound) interact with the tiger's roar (*Ooommm*). The yang sensations of the dragon (including gross tension) can interact with the smooth, pleasant yin sensations of the docile tiger. Sensations of light (the dragon) can merge or interact with sensations of darkness (the tiger).
3. Eventually the dragon and tiger will mate. This may bring the purified inner yang out of the tiger and the purified inner yin out of the dragon.
4. Proceed with formal Kan and Li meditation.

# INVOKING
# THE THREE PURE ONES

The Invocation of the Three Pure Ones is a practice that draws upon Lingbao Taoism and perhaps Zhang Dao-Ling's Religious Taoism (Tao-chiaou) as well. The practice includes purification, ceremony, and white magic, and thus it might appeal to those adepts with an interest in ancient Chinese culture. By personifying energies, the practice makes a connection to the archetypal dream worlds of the unconscious; for this reason it serves as a powerful lead-up to the Kan and Li formulas.

The Three Pure Ones are energies that arise from the Pole Star, though they are also said to arise from the stars, sun, and moon. Successful connection to the Three Pure Ones provides an antidote to the contraction and limitation caused by the Three Worms. Unfortunately, cultural differences between our Western Christianity-based culture and ancient Chinese folklore can make a connection to the Three Pure Ones difficult or implausible. Westerners are likely to have little understanding of an emperor or sovereign, although they may be able to relate to an archetypal king. Therefore the student needs to be flexible with this deep connection. To this we offer the following advice:

In general terms, the Pure Ones represent delicate, fine, and pleasurable energies that have the power to open and dilate the various blockages of the three tan tiens (fig. 4.5). Therefore in your meditation you should specifically identify the nature of the chi that is able to repeatedly and consistently do this. However, since every meditation is different and the perceived qualities of energies are ever changing, even this level of identification can be problematic. Nevertheless, persist! The key point to remember is that the Pure Ones are pleasurable, delicate, light, and pure. They can be regarded as highly purified fuel or energy that has the power to combat the Three Worms.

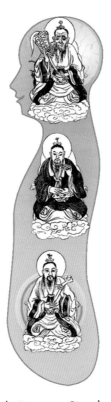

Fig. 4.5. Jade Emperor, Cinnabar Sovereign,
and Sovereign King opening the three tan tiens

## Invocation of the Three Pure Ones

1. Tune in to the Pole Star by becoming aware of the high-pitched sound coming from the heavens. Focus this sound as high as you can above the body onto one point. Initially this point will be close to the body but later far beyond it into the universe. Likewise allow the scalp to connect to this sensation.

2. Become aware of the first Pure One—Taiyi, the Jade Emperor, who opens the Crystal Palace. The Jade Emperor is associated with the stars and the firmament. The quality of its energy is close to the frequency and chi of the Pole Star, so the student may perceive an

extremely delicate high-frequency vibration. Its color can be white to violet, and the sound is a high-pitched *Eeeee* sound. This is somewhat similar to the dragon sound described elsewhere in this text. At times this frequency and sound is so soft that it just melts into a soothing light.

This energy is akin to the energy of the Great Spirit and corresponds to the Holy Spirit in Christianity. An overwhelming sense of awe and humility can occur along with activation of all the positive emotions. Delicate pulsing or fluttering of this energy may also occur. It focuses on the Crystal Palace and Jade Pillow and one finds the blissful release of the space between the base of the skull and the first cervical vertebra (atlas).

Relating to a Jade Emperor may be difficult for the aspiring adept. Emperors throughout history have been notoriously corrupt and easily influenced by self-serving officials. Examples include: Ming Chongzhen, who hung himself to end the Ming dynasty (1644), and Empress Dowager Cixi in the Qing dynasty (1835–1908), who had a reputation as a despot and villain. Therefore delve into your own dream world and subconscious to find a personality or God worthy of great power and status. If you are unable to connect with total purity, you may choose to connect with a younger emperor who in years to come will be worthy of this title. It may be a younger lady or man who contains the purity but requires a few more years of cultivation before fully achieving divine status.

3. Next, tune in to the frequency of Lao-tzu, the Cinnabar Sovereign who opens the Scarlet Palace—the heart tan tien. This is energy of a lower frequency than the Jade Emperor, yet it is just as refined. Its power has the ability to open the heart and combat the hold of the middle worm (see below). Its color is red; it's often felt as a light, smooth, and warm vapor. The association with love and respect is immediate. Finding such a personality or God is going to be unique to each individual adept. For some this may be symbolized

by the Christ or Buddha. One may also choose a specific ascended immortal.

4. The third Pure One is the Sovereign King who opens the Cinnabar Field.[3] The Sovereign King opens the lower tan tien and is often associated with a yellow color. The feelings here may be more watery and sexual in nature. The sound frequency takes on a somewhat lower vibration and can be described as the inner *Ooommm* sound, and here again there is overlap with and similarity to the tiger's sound. However, please note that the nature of this energy is so refined that it is a blend of the most purified energies that resonate with the lower tan tien. So while the energy can be described as watery and sexual, its quality is so much more pure than that. Like primordial energy—the energy before differentiation into yin and yang—the Sovereign King is similar to the substance of Wu Chi before the Big Bang! If you wish to connect to a personality or God from your dream consciousness, remember that this character is a little closer to the earth and should reflect this. This Pure One has the ability to release blockages around the sacrum, the groin, and the lumbar and lower thoracic spine.

## CORRESPONDENCES OF THE THREE PURE ONES

| NAME | YU HUANG JADE EMPEROR | LAO-TZU OLD PHILOSOPHER | TAO CHUN SOVEREIGN KING |
|---|---|---|---|
| Sects | Jade (Preexistence) | Lingbao | Shanqing |
| Energy | Pearly White | Red/Warm | Blue/Cool |
| Region | Head | Heart | Loins |
| Domain | Heaven | Earth | Humanity |
| Time | Present | Future | Past |
| Trinity | Shen | Chi | Ching |

# EXPELLING THE THREE WORMS (DEATH BRINGERS)

*Slay the Three Guards and ascend to the Ten Regions*
LAO-TZU[4]

In all phenomena beyond the unity state, there will always be the world of opposites. For each yang phenomenon there will be a yin phenomenon. The yang phenomena draw us to immortality and godlike status. Immortals do not require food, breath, or water. Yin desires include earthly pleasures such as solidity, sex, entertainment, and death. These yin qualities are not necessarily wrong or evil; they simply represent the other side of our dual nature.

Perfection in realizing the Tao is a slow and carefully graduated process. If our body and mind were to instantaneously become totally open and immortal-like, we would go mad. Instead, contraction and limitation represent an intermediate status between Heaven and Earth. For the Taoists, the Three Worms represented the need for contraction: they continuously reported to the Three Pure Ones the status of energy within the adept. They released when the entire being was ready to do so. This dynamic may be seen as a conflict, but it should ideally be regarded as a competitive approach to transcendence.

The Three Worms are the yin manifestations of the Three Pure Ones: instead of being made of chi and light, they are made of more material essences. They are described as being actual parasites that create disease, aging, and consequently premature death. Hence their alternate name of the Death Bringers.

The Three Worms[5] or monsters[6] also correspond to the three tan tiens (fig. 4.6) as follows.

*Ake (Peng Ju)* works on the upper tan tien and causes cravings of the external five senses—especially visual, auditory, olfactory, and taste cravings. It ages the head with

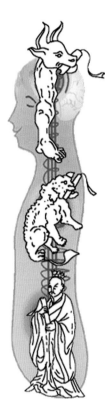

Fig. 4.6. The Three Worms correspond to the defilement of the three tan tiens.

deafness, blindness, loss of teeth, and wrinkles. Peng Ju in its external form is described as a one-legged, horned bull without a torso.

**Zuozi (Peng Zhi)** affects the heart predominantly, causing confusion in the mind and shen, which leads to a saddened heart. Peng Zhi is described as a mangy dog with an ugly head.

**Jixi (Peng Jiaou)** affects the lower tan tien and results in excessive fixated sexual desire with loss of semen and menses. It is described as a wayward priest.

Taoist physiology also includes some religious ideas; it is said that bad choices and unwise actions empower the Death Bringers, leading to disease and premature death.[7]

Meditation with the Three Worms

1. Begin this meditation with the Inner Smile. Then become aware of the knots and blockages that are closing down the three tan tiens. These knots and blockages correspond to defilements.

2. Use your imagination to create a multisensory impression of the Three Worms, giving shape to these defilements.

3. Create an inner dialogue with the Death Bringers: argue that your name needs to be transferred from the "Book of Death" to the "Book of Eternal (or Long) Life."

4. Part of slaying these three monsters is to rid the body of the Nine Worms described in the table below.[8] Visualize tightness in these areas as manifestations of attachment and disfigurement by the corresponding worms. Remove these worms with the radiant energy of the Three Pure Ones.

### LOCATION OF THE NINE WORMS[9]

| ACUPUNCTURE POINT | ANATOMY | WORM TYPE |
|---|---|---|
| GV 16 feng fu | C1 Base of skull | Prostrating Worm |
| BL 10 tian zhu | C1–2 1.5 cun lateral to midline | Dragon Worm |
| GV 13 tao dao | T1 (spine process of) | White Worm |
| GV 11 shen dao | T5 (spine process of) | Flesh Worm |
| GV 6 ji zhong | T11 (spine process of) | Green Worm |
| GV 5 xuan shu | L1(spine process of) | Worm of Hindrance |
| GV 4 ming men | L2 (spine process of) | Lung Worm |
| GV 3 yang guan | L4 (spine process of) | Stomach Worm |
| GV 1 chang qiang | Tip of coccyx | Golden Scale Bug |

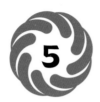

# The Greatest Kan and Li Formulas

*All methods end in quietness. This marvelous magic cannot be fathomed. But when the practice is started, one must press on from the obvious to the profound, from the coarse to the fine . . . and the end of the practice must be One.*

LU DONG-PIN[1]

The formulas of Greatest Kan and Li practice, which are included below, were passed down from Master Yi Eng. While it is important for practitioners to keep the integrity of these meditations in terms of their order, components, and goals, adepts do have a degree of flexibility. An experienced practitioner practicing alone can vary the order and even skip formulas or complete them partially before moving on to the next one. The continual theme of this text is that it is important to learn the formulas as they were originally taught, but it is also important to be flexible with them when they have been mastered, so that the meditation can be fluid and spontaneous.

All the formulas start with the gross or a fragment and take us to the fine and the whole. Each method will ultimately blend in with the others according to your unique personality and history. Each practice is accompanied by commentary from the authors, which explains the goals of the practice as well as advice on fine points of execution. The practices are also accompanied by frequently asked questions that have been raised during Universal Healing Tao workshops.

#  Connecting to the Two Poles

## Activating the Cranial and Sacral Pumps

The essentials of this practice have been developed in the Iron Shirt and Healing Love practices. The technique helps to open the crown by vibrating the bones at the sutures; it is then possible to project the pearl/soul/spirit out. Basically, the procedure assists in activating the cranial and sacral pumps, which are needed in the Alignment of Three Triangles, below.

The practice is similar to the Greater Kan and Li formula for spiraling through the crown and the feet (perineum) to set up Vertical and Earthly Flight. However, this time we extend beyond the earth and the imagined solar system to connect to the Pole Stars. In the original formulas set up by Yi Eng we did not include the South Celestial Pole, but through our global teachings we have realized the importance of connecting to both (fig. 5.1). Practitioners in the Northern Hemisphere connect to the Pole Star (Polaris) above the crown and Sigma Octanis (Polaris Australis) below the earth, while those in the Southern Hemisphere connect to Sigma Octanis above the crown and Polaris below.

## Connecting to the Pole Star above the Crown

1. Form another pearl and settle it in the perineum.
2. Move the pearl around the Microcosmic Orbit and let it gather momentum.

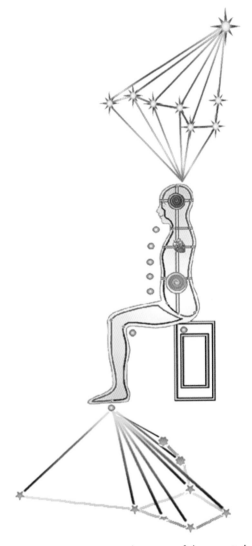

Fig. 5.1. Connecting to the stars of the two Poles

3. Slow it down and let it rest in the crown.

4. Activate the cranial pump (look up, clench the teeth and jaw, sink chin and sternum, clench the fists, tighten the buttocks, and pull up the sexual organs).

5. Exhale and shoot the pearl through the crown, extending it many body-lengths above you.

6. Swallow saliva upward as you feel the earth force come up to you.

7. Exhale and completely relax any muscles you have tensed. You must be able to totally release all body tension so that the chi can flow easily through the pumps and throughout the body. Work toward activating these pumps through structural alignment and mental focus only.

8. Draw the yang energy from the Pole Star into the Crystal Room and other tan tiens. Merge this experience with that of the Third Eye.

## ❂ Connecting to the Pole Star beneath the Earth

1. Shoot the pearl down the legs, many body-lengths into the ground, and then beyond the earth to the Pole Star beneath. Connect with its more yin nature.

2. Create a pakua around the pearl.

3. Extend the Thrusting Routes and Belt Routes to the body/bodies in and beneath the earth.

4. Gather in the middle of the toes, in the tan tiens, and at the mid-eyebrow. You may then merge the Third Eye with the earth plane experience.

## Commentary

**Goals:** The goals for this practice are many. The first is to extend consciousness beyond self. This is in keeping with our broad concept of the Wu Wei experience, whereby we must first embrace everything before we can perceive the "nothing." This is particularly true from the perspective of geography/space.

The second goal is to assist in aligning the body so that all the forces are in unison and working together. This can be understood as aligning the earth force with the heavenly force and the body's internal energies, or as harmonizing the resident spirits within the body. The dragon spirit works with the spirit that exists above the crown (the highest soul) to reach the Pole Star above. The tiger spirit works with the earth soul beneath the feet to extend consciousness to the opposite Pole Star. The spirits in the head, heart, abdomen, and behind the knees all serve to align the body with these vertical forces.

The third goal is to receive pure energies from the Pole Star. As early as the Han era, Taoists believed that the Pole Star encompassed the unitive experience. Ge Hong says, "The One resides at the North Pole . . . dragons and tigers are lined up on guard."[2] In the Universal Healing Tao, the Pole Star is not only the gateway to an experience of the One; it also emits a violet healing light that has a remarkable healing effect and a specific resonance with the bones of the body. The Pole Star beneath is usually felt as more yin.

**Advice:** The connection to the Pole Stars can be achieved by means other than shooting a pearl. Adepts can also use the spiraling technique to follow the natural wave pattern of a vortex. One vortex connects the Crystal Room to the heavens and the Pole Star above. The second vortex connects the perineum or feet to the earth and the Pole Star beneath the earth.

You can also use the spirits to assist you: the heavenly soul can ride the dragon and use the high-pitched *Eeeeee* sound to transport your mind to Polaris. Likewise you can use the roaring *Ooommm* of the tiger's sound with the assistance of the earth soul to access the connection to Polaris Australis. (Obviously, if you are practicing in the Southern Hemisphere, the stars are reversed.) The Pole Star above you can connect to the whole crown but should specifically connect to the Ba Hui point (at the midpoint above the apex of the ears). The lower pole connects to the tip of the coccyx or the soles of the feet, depending whether you are sitting cross-legged or standing.

The connection to the Pole Star doesn't necessarily have to occur at the start of your Kan and Li session. You can connect faintly at the start and solidify that connection later after some coupling and steaming.

## Frequently Asked Questions

**Question:** I have trouble connecting to Polaris. I have tried all the techniques of shooting pearls, spiraling, and following the mythical creatures' sounds but to no avail. Sometimes I can see the Pole Star but I have no physical connection to it! What can I do?

**Response:** You may be attempting this meditation too early in your meditation session. If your body is too tight and/or your intellectual mind is overactive, then failure is likely. You must spend more time with your warm-ups until you are really settled. The power and ability comes from being settled and not from being overzealous and premature. Extending consciousness far away is no easy feat. You may also seek assistance by attending a class and letting the teacher guide you. Alternatively, arrange time away from your work-a-day life so you have lots of space and time for practice. You may need to set up a framework, much like a retreat, where the burden of decision-making and food preparation is taken away from you.

## COUPLING IN THE HEART

We established the cauldron earlier in the navel, then in the solar plexus; now we place it at the heart center. Note that the same channels (Left, Right, and Middle Thrusting; Conception and Governing) are used as in the Lesser and Greater Kan and Li practices. You can set up the lower tan tien cauldron and then proceed to the solar plexus cauldron. Finally, once the area around the diaphragm is steamed and the channels have opened, then couple at the heart. All three cauldrons can be firing at the same time or you can focus on one in particular.

## Establishing the Cauldron in the Heart

1. Collect the warm energies of the hands, arms, shoulders, upper chest, heart, neck, and head in the Crystal Room.

2. Add the cold/watery energies of the earth, legs, and hips to the perineum collection point.

3. Move the hot/fiery energies from the adrenals, thymus, and heart up to the Crystal Room. Use a vortex to add the heavenly force.

4. Use another vortex to add the earth force to the cold/watery energies in the perineum.

5. Move the hot/fire energy from the Crystal Room to the solar plexus via the Left Thrusting Channel and/or the back Governing Vessel (fig. 5.2). Simultaneously move the cold/water energy from the

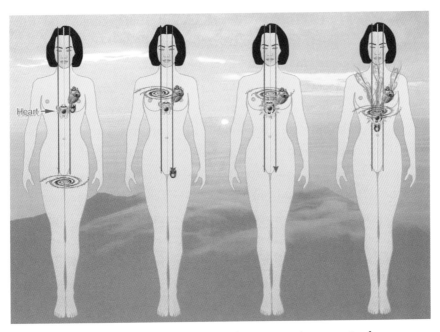

Fig. 5.2. Coupling in the heart involves moving hot energies from the Crystal Palace down the Left Thrusting Channel and cool energies up from the perineum via the Right Thrusting Channel.

perineum to the throat center via the Right Thrusting Channel and/or the Conception Vessel.

6. Sink the sternum, round the scapulae, sink the chin, arch the sacrum/coccyx. Move the heart toward the spine. This will assist in the coupling/cupping process.

7. Bring the fire energies and the water energies into the Middle Thrusting Channel and then to the cauldron in the heart center. Begin coupling.

8. Use the rhythm of the breath, the pulse, or other methods to fan the fire.

9. Begin the steaming process.

## Commentary

**Goal:** The purpose of this practice is similar to those described in previous Kan and Li texts. The aim is to combine disparate energies and make them into one; this is part of the reversal of the Taoist creation theory as we march back from multiplicity to unity. However, some details are different, because we are now coupling in the heart.

The first goal is to obtain a more refined fire and water. Each time we move up a cauldron within the body, the two opposite energies are more pure. They can also be described as more true. Remember that when we heat water in the lower cauldron, much of the steam can also be used to heat the solar plexus cauldron. The steam, which contains the heat from the firing, ultimately condenses to form more purified water. Thus we go through the process of extracting pure fire out of tainted water and pure water out of tainted fire. Of course, impure fire and water will still be gathered from areas of the body as we continue the coupling process. But ultimately, once the whole body is open and all tension released, we can discover pure yin and yang. Once we have pure yin and yang, they can be mated to form the Golden Elixir.

The second goal is to impregnate our fetus with the Shen. So far we have added the Hun (ethereal soul of the liver) in Lesser Kan and Li, and the Yi (the intention spirit of the spleen) in Greater Kan and Li. Now we add the Shen from the heart. Another way of saying this is that we couple Kan and Li in an environment of pure love. This bliss has a profound effect on the development of our embryo. It allows the principle of love and compassion to enter into our reunification. The ultimate aim, of course, is to merge all the nine spirits into the spiritual fetus before it is ready to leave the body.

The third goal is to allow the coupling to clear the chest cavity of knots, tension, and blocked channels. This optimizes our health and bodily functioning.

**Advice:** Opening the third eye is an important aspect to success. If you can then merge the coupling process in the heart with the visions in the third eye, then the coupling is most efficient and transformative. The aim is to superimpose the tactile sensations and energetic awareness of the region of the heart onto the visual sensations of the third eye.

Note that hot energies can be gathered from areas of tension anywhere, and you don't have to stick exactly to the formulas described above. If the coupling is already set up, these hot energies can be added directly to the fire instead of going via the Crystal Room.

## Frequently Asked Questions

**Question:** I seem to be able to visualize or imagine the coupling but do not feel much. I feel that I'm missing out on something. What else can I do?

**Response:** Excessive visualization at the expense of the other senses is occasionally a problem. Liu I-Ming is critical of excessive visualizations, as this is a distraction to the ultimate purpose.[3] The aim is to fuse all senses and return to the primordial, which is beyond visualization. Therefore it is important to utilize all the senses. Coupling is a whole body and mind activity, involving the empty force, breath-holding, swallowing saliva, and sexual desire in addition to the senses. To start, you can just work with the coming together of the sounds of the tiger and the dragon (*Ooommm* and *Eeeeee*). Use the portals of sound to regulate the intensity; listen above the crown to increase yang, and listen below the perineum to increase yin.

Next, try grounding yourself in the kinesthetic sense by feeling the breath and the pulsing in the heart and arteries. Occasionally massage your body to keep away from the monkey mind, which prefers thought and visualization as its primary vehicles of awareness. Self-massage can also arouse sexual desire. Don't forget to roll the eyes back. Finally, use your hands to guide the chi: this will improve your kinesthetic sense and facilitate coupling.

**Question:** You mentioned breath-holding, sexual desire, the empty force, and swallowing saliva in your response to the last question. Can you explain again how they are involved in the coupling process?

**Response:** Unfortunately, the rewards of meditation lie at the extremes of breath patterns. Most of the chi that you require lies at the end of your breath. Breath-holding occurs spontaneously as the mind gets lost in the bliss of the energies perceived. However, breath-holding is initially surrounded with fear. It is the inner sexual pleasure that can take you through this fear and pain; willpower alone will not suffice. So you push through the boundaries of the everyday breathing existence and enter into the embryo's domain. The embryo does not breathe, but it does swallow saliva and amniotic fluid!

The empty force is a key component of coupling. As the abdomen gets sucked in, more internal channels open up. The suction force enables the opposite energies to intermingle. At times, you may make stridor-type sounds through a partially closed larynx rather than breathing normally.

In addition to the empty force, there are also sustained periods of breath-holding (apnea) associated with the packing breath (bearing down) and high intra-abdominal pressures. These often result in bursts of inner light and the opening of consciousness to new dimensions.

Swallowing saliva is also a feature of coupling. This reflex of swallowing occurs in fetal existence and in the realm of no-breath. It is not performed through the thought of the monkey mind but happens by itself. When this reflex is activated, the adept should not interfere with it but should go with the process.

**Question:** You mentioned the third eye being very important in coupling. Can you explain this further?

**Response:** The third eye facilitates the complicated coupling procedure in many ways. Mostly, it enables the body and mind to coordinate the many elements involved (i.e., empty force, sexual desire, breath-holding, and juxtaposing the diametric opposite energies of Kan and Li). While the monkey mind can only focus on one aspect at a time, the third eye enables all these procedures to happen at once. The mind just needs to observe rather than interfere. Observation alone is enough to coordinate everything.

Opening the third eye also helps broaden consciousness outside of oneself, which is paramount to perceiving that you and the universe are one.

**Question:** I seemed to be able to couple in the lower tan tien and solar plexus but have had difficulty firing the cauldron in the heart. What else can I do?

**Response:** Do not commence coupling until the body is sufficiently open and loose to allow it. If you start too early, then you may get coupling that occurs for a few minutes, but it will soon peter out.

You may have some blockages in the chest preventing the coupling. This is not uncommon. Perhaps allow yourself more time for the practice. Alternatively, maybe practice only the Lesser and Greater Kan and Li formulas if you are rushed and busy with your work schedule. When you have time, go through the Fusion practices in *Cosmic Fusion* and *Fusion of the Eight Psychic Channels*.* Working the Belt and Thrusting Channels in the chest is ideal preparation for Greatest Kan and Li. Spinal Cord Cutting is also terrific for removing blockages in the thoracic and cervical spine.

**Question:** How intense should the coupling be? Sometimes I hear other students making lots of noises. They also seem to sweat a lot and generate much heat. They also see lots of lights!

**Response:** Please remember that coupling is similar to making love to your partner: some couples make a lot of noise while others are quiet. There is no right or wrong way. Many women state that the process is a quieter affair for them with less tension, pressure, and noises. There are times when my coupling is more passive and quiet. Certainly for many practitioners, the process becomes more yin as the years pass. Usually, the more delicate the more powerful! So the answer is that both loud and quiet coupling can occur and neither is incorrect. However, forcing any part of it is wrong. By the same token, if the student is too passive and avoiding intensity and pain (good, pleasurable pain), then that is not right either.

Seeing lights is nice but is something that should not distract the practitioner. The desire to see lights and have some sort of psychedelic experience is the wrong intention. Your true intention should be to experience stillness. Therefore, if your meditation is not so intense, but is very gentle and produces the desired result, then you are doing well. Please don't be sidetracked into transient pleasures of the individual senses: we are after a whole mind-body experience of nothingness!

**Question:** How long should one couple for?

**Response:** Again, there is no right or wrong answer here. Coupling can

---

*See Mantak Chia, *Cosmic Fusion* (Rochester, Vt.: Destiny Books, 2007) and *Fusion of the Eight Psychic Channels* (Rochester, Vt.: Destiny Books, 2008).

occur for as long as you like! The body and mind will naturally become satiated with this intense activity and there will be periods of valley orgasms or bliss that last for varying periods of time. Sometimes the urge to couple will occur again. In each series of couplings the energies become more pure. There is a blissful drift from coupling disparate energies to an experience of the Primordial Force. After each episode of coupling new dimensions will appear. These new dimensions will again need to be coupled and merged in the march toward the unitive experience.

##  Steaming Formula

1. To fan the fire of the cauldron, use bellows breathing until the energy begins to boil.
2. Establish a pulse at the cauldron and use this pulse to maintain the heat of the cauldron.
3. Turn the senses into the cauldron and stir with the eyes.
4. As steam comes out of the cauldron, direct it to the glands, organs, lymph, nerves, endocrine system, and channels, including the Microcosmic Orbit, Thrusting Channels, Belt Routes, Great Bridge, and Regulator Channels. Also direct steam to the Crystal Room (see fig. 5.3 on page 132).
5. Be mindful of the condensation of steam and the dripping of purified Kan. Especially watch for dripping from the Crystal Room. The drops that come from the mammillary body are special. These droplets can form a pool in the heart, solar plexus, or perineum. This purified Kan or pure yin is essential to forming the embryo.

## Commentary

**Goal:** The purpose of steaming is twofold. The first is to cleanse the organs and channels. This means we remove any congestion that exists in the region of the organ. Congestion feels like unpleasant prickly heat or

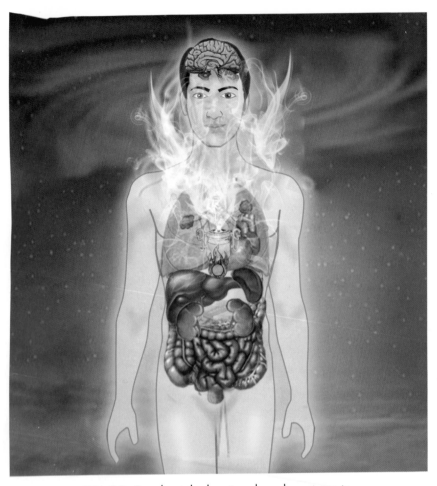

Fig. 5.3. Couple at the heart and produce steam to
extract pure yin essence from the organs.

cold. Opened channels feel smooth while blocked channels feel tense and
tight, like knots.

Secondly, the essence of the organ is captured from the steam and
used for its pure yin or yang essence. This essence drips into the cauldron
and is one step closer to preparation of the Golden Elixir. As we progress
through the Kan and Li series and into Sealing of the Five Senses, we
attain the ability to steam and cleanse parts of the body that were previously unreachable or not known. This includes parts of the brain includ-

ing the mamillary bodies, thalamus, hypothalamus, optic and olfactory nerves, memory center, and so on.

**Advice:** Steaming is a sensation that arises above the coupling; it includes both a wet heat and a fine-frequency vibration. Students have various experiences, but a common one is a pleasant warm and wet sensation that has an immediate opening effect. This force cleanses and removes inner blockages or adhesions. When the steam condenses, it gathers the essence of the solid organ that is cleansed.

In the language of External Alchemy, steaming extracts the yin from cinnabar as mercury (true yin or mercury), which then flows down into the cauldron. It extracts the yang from the lead as silver (true lead or yin), which can then combine with mercury to become gold. The difference between Inner and External Alchemy is that in Inner Alchemy purified yang energy *becomes* the fire: the fire is not only a facilitator for formation of the prima materia, but it also contributes of itself to forming that material.

Furthermore, steam can be used to heat the cauldron(s) above it. In the Greatest Kan and Li, steam from the lower cauldron and solar plexus tan tien can be used to heat the heart cauldron. In other words, as we progress the steaming, we use a more yin and delicate fire. We make the Li more yin, which is described in the *Dragon Tiger Classic* as extracting the yang out of yin. The yang tiger is extracted from lead (the kidneys). Alternatively, we extract the yang straight line out of the trigram Kan to produce Heaven (yang-yang-yang), and extract the yin broken lines out of the trigram Li to produce Earth (yin-yin-yin). Hence we can steam the heart as representative of fire to produce yin essence.

This is a convoluted understanding of Internal Alchemy, and it has the potential to cause misunderstanding. For those who find this discussion perplexing, just stick to using the steam to cleanse and purify. That is, use the steam to open channels, remove inner energetic knots (worms), and distill pure yin out of organs.

## Frequently Asked Questions

**Question:** I do not feel any steam. What am I doing wrong?

**Response:** If the steaming sensation isn't occurring, relax a little more so that the coupling is not so intense or rigid. Also relax around the cauldron.

Sometimes a student may be steaming and simply not realizing it. Coupling definitely makes the whole body hot. Most people sweat with the process as well. You can probably see how steaming fits into this picture. Steaming can vary in its sensations. Some experience it as a delicate dissolution of tension above the cauldron. Others experience it as a sensation halfway between water and fire—a combination of the two energies. Others visualize the steam in their mind's eye. Everyone is different in the way that they sense and interpret the internal happenings around the imagined cauldron. So don't be too hard on yourself if your sensations are different from others. Just bear the goals in mind.

If you are experiencing a loosening or opening, then one aim is achieved. If you obtain a more pleasant combined sensation above the cauldron, then the second goal is achieved.

**Question:** I have difficulty directing the steam. What should I do?

**Response:** Whenever difficulties occur it is best to pause momentarily: really relax and sink more. Lessen the willpower and expectation! Allow the meditation to unfold naturally and spontaneously. It is likely that you are forcing the process.

Another option is to drop down a cauldron and steam from a lower site. Remember that the lower cauldron is made of clay and the solar plexus cauldron made of iron. Both can withstand a more chaotic fire and are therefore easier to control, allowing you to direct the steam more easily to the desired place. Therefore don't become fixated on using only one cauldron. Each cauldron has different functions. As we rise up, the fire and water must be purified in order to handle the purer energies.

Alignment of the Three Triangles

The three double triangles that we align in this exercise include: the Crystal Room and the chin bone; the sternum and xiphisternum; and the bony pelvic inlet and the sacrum.

This formula can be used as a warm-up, during coupling, or post-coupling.

1. **The upper triangle** (Crystal Room and chin bone): Pull the jaw/chin back toward the cervical vertebrae, thus straightening the Jade Pillow. Gently stretch your neck up and open C7 to align them with the crown (fig. 5.4). This also aligns the Crystal Room (pituitary

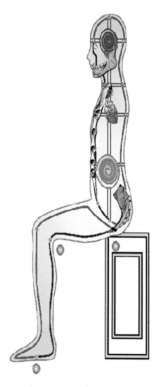

Fig. 5.4. Alignment of the Three Triangles:
The Crystal Palace/mandible, the sternum/xiphisternum,
and the bony pelvic inlet/sacrum

gland, pineal gland, fornix, mammillary body) with the lower triangles.

2. **The middle triangle** (sternum and xiphisternum): Allow the sternum to move down by softly sinking the chest. This motion moves the heart center and sternum back and aligns the middle triangle with the sacrum/coccyx triangle below and the Crystal Room above.

3. **The lower triangle** (pelvic bones and sacrum): Arch the sacrum and tilt the coccyx down. This will align the sacrum to the upper and middle triangles and the coccyx to the earth.

4. If you are practicing this meditation on its own, collect the energy in the lower tan tien and Turn the Wheel. Ideally, you would Turn the Wheel 360 times back to front and then 360 times front to back.

Work on the Alignment of the Three Triangle Forces as a separate practice until you are comfortable with it. Note that the bones of the three triangle forces are themselves bi-triangular in shape (Crystal Palace/chin, sternum/xiphoid process, and pelvic inlet/sacrum). Triangle and pointed bones are able to project and attract energy more efficiently than round or flat bones.

When you align the three triangle forces, it is easy to see that they create a kind of arrow—a trajectory upward to the North Star and downward to the earth. Thus the physical body and its varied energies and technology become an efficient machine for attracting different forces, and for projecting and fusing those energies between Heaven and Earth. The practitioner develops himself/herself into a powerful instrument capable of attuning itself with great precision to its purest source.

## Commentary

**Goals:** The aim of this meditation is to align the three regions of the body and their associated bony components. In some respects, this practice is similar to merging the three tan tiens, although the tan tiens do not include the bones. Using the combination of triangular bones and the tan tien regions nearby creates a unique vibration and directional flow that assists in opening deep internal channels.

Although aligning and merging the three tan tiens is a basic UHT practice, it requires ongoing work and development, like all basic practices. At this level we really draw upon the Three Pure Ones, who arise via the North Star and represent energies that come from the three large stars beyond it. The upper tan tien receives and radiates chi from the Crystal Palace. This chi represents purified Shen. The middle tan tien receives and emits purified chi. The lower tan tien works and glows with true Ching Chi. The corresponding deities (while they vary according to the various Taoist sects) were discussed in chapter 4.

The bony component adds a new dimension to this meditation. The frequency of bone vibration is different than the vibration of the tan tien. It has a higher pitch and perhaps a white color. The bones also assist a unidirectional flow from the Pole Star above to the earth below. This flow assists in removing residual tension and blockages in the current stage of the adept's meditation.

**Advice:** Always begin by being confident in your knowledge of the specific anatomy. In the upper triangle, the Crystal Palace is an imaginary crystal prism that extends from the pineal gland to the pituitary gland. It houses the third ventricle, the thalamus, and the hypothalamus. Don't forget that the thalamus extends laterally and looks like two eggs with the smaller conical end facing posteriorly. The chin—the lower part of the upper triangle—extends from the ears to the chin and comprises the lower jaw.

For the middle triangle, the sternum extends from the sternal notch at the bottom of the throat down to the xiphisternum. The xiphisternum (the lower part of the middle triangle) is triangular in shape and provides a unidirectional aspect to the flow of chi. The xiphisternum is easily palpated at the superior aspect of the solar plexus.

At the lower triangle, the sacrum and coccyx form the triangular posterior aspect of the pelvis and the remnant of a tail. This time we don't exactly involve the lower tan tien but the region below it and above the perineum. This energy is more associated with sexual (Ching) rather than the lower tan tien, which blends abdominal organ energy as well.

## Frequently Asked Questions

**Question:** Can you explain the difference between the Three Minds into One Mind meditation and this Alignment of the Three Triangles? They seem very similar.

**Response:** These two practices are very similar as they both include the three tan tiens. However, there are a few differences. First of all, the lower triangular force is just below the lower tan tien. Secondly, the bony component alters the vibrational sum of these areas, so that they are different than the tan tiens themselves. The heart has a certain softness and warmth to it, the brain has a certain muddy, mushy quality, and the region below the lower tan tien has a certain silk-like quality. Bone, on the other hand, has a high-pitched quality. In this formula you blend the qualities to come up with something new.

Finally, there is a directional component. The three tan tiens merge within the body and do not have a sense of flow. The three triangles, however, create a strong flow from the Pole Star above to the earth and the Pole Star beneath.

## Connecting the Cranial Bones to the Stars

In this meditation, we connect the bones of the skull to the stars. Northern Hemisphere practitioners connect to the seven stars of the Big Dipper and the North Star, while Southern Hemisphere practitioners connect to the Southern Cross and its two pointers.

## ☺ Northern Hemisphere: Big Dipper and Pole Star Cranial Connections

1. Connect the left mastoid bone with Dubhe (the tip of the cup) (fig. 5.5).
2. Connect the right mastoid bone with Merak (the base of the cup closest to Polaris).

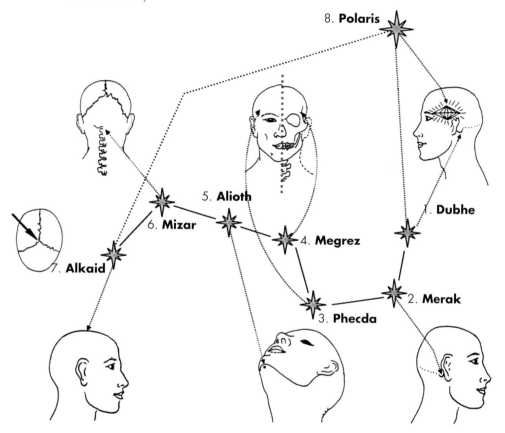

1. **Dubhe:** The Pivot of the Sky, left mastoid, wood/Jupiter/Thursday (near west)

2. **Merak:** Revolver, right mastoid, water/Mercury/Wednesday

3. **Phecda:** The Rotator of the Sky, right temple and cheekbone, earth/Saturn/Saturday

4. **Megrez:** Leveling Light, left temple and cheekbone, water/Mercury/Wednesday

5. **Alioth:** Balancing Light, chin, fire/Mars/Tuesday (near north)

6. **Mizar:** Generating Light, base of the skull, metal/Venus/Friday

7. **Alkaid:** Harmonizing Light, crown G.P.M., water/Mercury/Wednesday

8. **Polaris:** Crystal Room (pineal, pituitary, thalamus)

Fig. 5.5. Craniofacial connections to the Big Dipper and Polaris

3. Connect the right temple and cheekbone with Phecda (the base of the cup closest to the handle).

4. Connect the left temple and cheekbone with Megrez (the tip of the cup closest to the handle).

5. Connect the chin with Alioth (the handle of dipper closest to cup).

6. Connect the base of the occiput with Mizar (the middle star of the handle of the dipper).

7. Connect the anterior fontanelle of the crown with Alkaid (the first star of the handle; furthest from the cup). This crown point is the junction of the frontal, parietal, and coronal sutures of the skull.

8. Connect the Crystal Room to Polaris.

## ❷ Southern Hemisphere: Craniofacial Connections to the Southern Cross and Pointers

As discussed earlier, there is no Taoist literature on connections for those practitioners south of the equator. My suggestion (Andrew Jan) is to use the Southern Cross and its two pointers, which together yield seven stars. These stars can then be connected to the same bones (and neural bodies) as the stars in the Northern Hemisphere.

1. Connect the anterior fontanelle of the crown (the junction of the frontal, parietal, and coronal sutures of the skull) to Alpha Crux (fig. 5.6).

2. Connect the chin with Epsilon Crux.

3. Connect the right temple and cheekbone with Delta Crux.

4. Connect the right mastoid bone with Beta Crux.

5. Connect the left mastoid bone with Beta Centauri.

6. Connect the left temple and cheekbone with Alpha Centauri.

7. Connnect the base of the occiput with Gamma Crux.

8. Connect the Crystal Room with Polaris Australis.

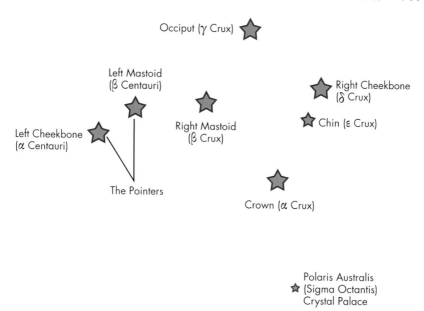

Fig. 5.6. Craniofacial connections to the Southern Cross
and its two pointers

## Commentary

**Goals:** The aim of this exercise is to make a connection between the various parts of the cranium and the Big Dipper/Southern Cross-Polaris complex. This connection offers many benefits.

The connection will often dissipate remnants of tension in the face and cranium. Having tension in the body is a continual reminder of the small self (microcosm); while such tension exists, there cannot be total merging of the microcosm with the macrocosm. Connecting any remnants of tension with solid stars somehow seems to assist in the dissolving of these blockages. The opening of various parts of the skull allows the channels of the face and cranium to open as well. The following vessels traverse the skull and face: Governing, Small Intestine, Gall Bladder, Stomach, Triple Warmer, Large Intestine, Bladder, and Conception Vessels.

The connections achieved in the formula orient the mind and body toward the Pole Star, a focal stillpoint around which all multiplicity rotates. The Three Pure Ones—including the Jade Emperor—reside there. By connecting to the Pole Star, the three tan tiens open and release. Furthermore, the Pole Star is said to generate a unique violet chi.

**Advice:** Making craniofacial connection to the Big Dipper (or Southern Cross and two pointers) and the Pole Stars is relatively straightforward. There are only two prerequisites. The first is that you are familiar with the respective constellations and the anatomy of the skull and face. The second is that you have sufficient depth in your meditation that the channels in the head region are at least partially open.

Spend some time stargazing. Use a constellation map to be precise with the names of each star. Try to view the Pole Star region at various times so that you get a real appreciation of the rotation of the constellations around that fixed point. Once the connection is made and you feel opening of the various craniofacial points, you can spin the stars. This has the effect of merging space and also time.

With regard to the depth of your meditation, there may be times when you can use this meditation as a warm-up before coupling. At other times the body may be a little tight; in this case you can couple for a while to open the craniofacial region before making the connections.

## Frequently Asked Questions

**Question:** Can I make connections to the pelvic region with the stars on the opposite pole?

**Response:** This is a good question. As we have said previously, the traditional teachings did not include the Polaris Australis or the Southern Cross. In those days, practitioners connected the earth to the coccyx, sacrum, and perineum. The force was yin and water-like. If you wish to connect your pelvic bones to something other than the earth, it may be better to connect the feet and lower part of the body to the twelve Earthly Branches. You could then connect the tip of your coccyx with the opposite Pole Star. If there is still some residual tension you could make star connections with the sitting bones (ischial tuberosities), iliac crests, or even the lesser trochanters. Use your own inventiveness.

**Question:** The Big Dipper and Southern Cross rotate around the Pole Stars. This makes alignment difficult, especially when the surrounding constellation is behind the Pole Star.

**Response:** Yes, the Big Dipper rotates around the Pole Star like an hour hand around the center of the clock. However, you can use your imagination to cross over the connections. Ultimately the aim is to have a twenty-four-hour connection. This is especially important if you are on retreat doing practice during the day and night. The connection thus becomes circular; with time you can dissolve these sequential connections into one.

 Connecting with the Heavenly Stems and Earthly Branches

### Connecting with the Ten Heavenly Stems

1. Begin by connecting to the five visible planets and their corresponding elements: Jupiter/wood, Mars/fire, Saturn/earth, Venus/metal, and Mercury/water. Link Jupiter to the right parietal bone, Mars to the frontal bone, Saturn to the center of the crown, Venus to the left parietal bone, and Mercury to the occipital bone. Keep this order as it maintains the Creation Cycle.

2. Assign each planet/element a yin and a yang phase to create a ten-day cycle. The first day of each element is yang and the second yin. In this way we can connect with time according to the five elements (Jupiter/wood: Jia, Yi; Mars/fire: Bing, Ding; Saturn/earth: Wu, Ji; Venus/metal: Geng, Xin; and Mercury/water: Ren, Gui).

3. Assign each stem a region of the firmament, such that the entire universe is covered in terms of space (see fig. 5.7 on page 144).

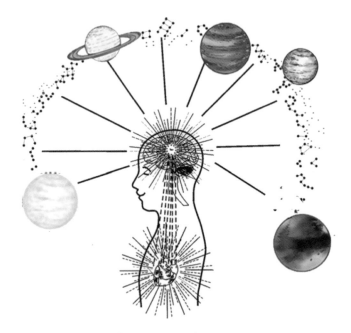

Fig. 5.7. The ten Heavenly Stems connect
to the five planets in a ten-day cycle.

## ❷ Connecting with the Twelve Earthly Branches

1. Connect to the twelve Earthly Branches by radiating out arcs of energy (or shooting pearls) from the sacrum and perineum, in much the same pattern as the anatomical nerves. Commence a new arc every 30 degrees, and number them from 1 to 12 (fig. 5.8).

2. Think of time as well as space. Imagine the earth spinning like a clock. Name each two-hour time period of the day as follows: Zi: 11 p.m.–1 a.m., Rat; Chou: 1–3 a.m., Buffalo; Yin: 3–5 a.m., Tiger; Mao: 5–7 a.m., Rabbit; Chen: 7–9 a.m., Dragon; Si: 9–11 a.m., Snake; Wu: 11 a.m.–1 p.m., Horse; Wei: 1–3 p.m., Goat; Shen: 3–5 p.m., Monkey; You: 5–7 p.m., Rooster; Xu: 7–9 p.m., Dog; and Hai: 9–11 p.m., Pig.

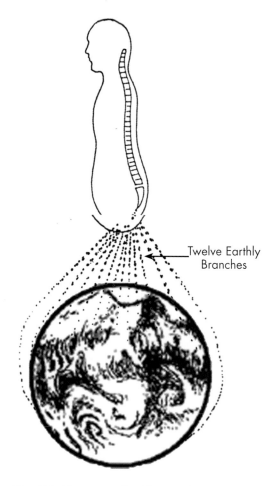

Fig. 5.8. The twelve Earthly Branches
make thirty-degree arcs around the earth.

## ☯ Conclusion

1. Connect the ten Heavenly Stems and twelve Earthly Branches with your mind, then merge them into one!
2. If practicing this meditation in isolation, collect the energy in the lower tan tien and Turn the Wheel. Ideally this is done 360 times back to front, then reversed the same number of times.

## Commentary

**Goals:** The purpose of the Heavenly Stems and Earthly Branches practice is first of all to understand that Earth comes from Heaven and that Earth is therefore the branch. The heavens stem from the Wu Wei. The second goal is to cover all aspects of time and space. This we do in several stages, first by connecting to the ten days of the Shang-era week, then by connecting to all parts of the day according to two-hour units. Next, we connect to the entire universe radiating out from the visible planets to cover all of the heavens. Then we connect to every corner of the globe by covering every thirty degrees of longitude. To realize the One, we must include all of space and time.

**Advice:** Find yourself a clear location where you can stargaze. Have access to information that lets you know the rising and setting times of each of the five visible planets and the moon. These days, you can easily purchase a cheap application for your mobile phone that will locate the planets exactly. This precision helps to support your meditation, because the actual sighting or locating of the planet will assist the meditative mind in connecting to that planet.

In your meditation, you can also connect the planets within the ecliptic (the plane that the sun and planets follow) to the solid and hollow organs. Yin represents the solid organs (liver, heart, spleen, lungs, kidneys), while yang represents the hollow organs (gallbladder, small intestine, stomach, large intestine, urinary bladder). Once you have made these connections, link to the universe beyond and the five-element distribution of stars. Note that according to some traditional Taoist theories, there exist five elemental stars that can be connected to via Polaris.

The Earthly Branches are simpler to connect with. You simply connect with sections of the earth marked by every thirty degrees of longitude. Once you have covered the entire globe, allow the earth to spin.

Ultimately, all of the days can be merged into one via the five-element planets and stars. Once the days have been merged, you can fuse the twelve two-hour units into one by covering the entire earth and allowing it to spin.

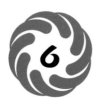

# Supplemental Practices

 ## Pulsating the Heart with the Aorta (Sun) and the Vena Cava (Moon)

1. Use the mind to follow the yin vena cava and yang aorta as they move the blood toward and away from the heart. The outflow (aorta) is hot and yang and is thus connected to the sun. The inflow (vena cava) is cool and yin and connects to the moon.

2. Collect the electricity from both sides of the head, neck, shoulders, upper chest, arms, and hands, and collect it in the heart (see fig. 6.1 on page 148). Feel the recharging of energy.

3. The kidneys act as step-up transformers of the energy in the lower branches of the aorta and vena cava; use your mind to direct the circulation of blood in the lower part of the legs up to the kidneys, then feel the two kidneys become electrically charged. Direct the energy back to the heart.

4. If practicing this meditation in isolation, collect the energy in the lower tan tien and Turn the Wheel. Ideally this is done 360 times back to front, then front to back for another 360 times.

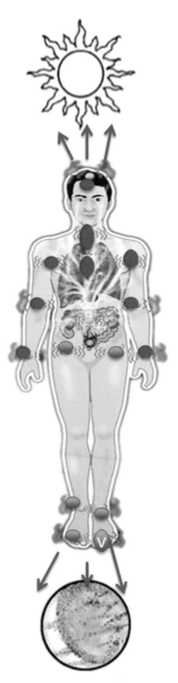

Fig. 6.1. Connecting the sun and moon to
the heart's hot outflow and cool inflow

## Commentary

**Goals:** The aim of this practice is to merge the pulsing of the body with the body's polar energies. The natural and mortal physiology is for heat (fire, Li, and yang energies) to accumulate in the upper half of the body while the bottom half remains cool. The aim of the practice is to gather these sensations prior to and during formal coupling. By gathering them one can dissipate tension and relieve blocked channels and congestion.

Pulsing was described as a warm-up in chapter 4. This is a further development of that practice; it prompts you to feel the suction of cool blood and chi with the aid of the kidneys. You can even add the sense of sound to this meditation and hear a *WOOOSH* as blood returns and an *MMMM* sound as it exits the heart. You may further choose to involve your whole body by using the sensations and imagery of riding a horse, for example. As your body rocks forward feel the warm, red, glowing chi. As your body rocks backward, feel the cooler more stagnant energy returning. The Kua is opened in the process, and the cooler Ching Chi and Kidney Chi flow freely. Alternatively, you can imagine yourself as a child or even a fetus listening to and feeling the pulses as a lullaby. The lullaby not only focuses the mind but dissolves tension and blockages as well.

**Advice:** While this meditation is listed as a formula for Greatest Kan and Li proper, it can also be used as a warm-up and a continuation of the Pulsing Exercise. However, it is useful after coupling has started as well. The student can use this meditation to assist in the gathering of the polar energies in order that they may be coupled. It is also helpful for those times when coupling has spontaneously ceased. The student can regroup, gather the polar energies, and commence self-intercourse again. Finally, this exercise can be carried out while coupling is in progress. This has the effect of fanning the fire.

Once you have identified the poles, don't leave them as they are. Either couple the two poles or Turn the Wheel to finish. As an extension of this practice, you can extend the venous phase to collect cool blood from the upper body and extend the arterial phase to encompass the lower limbs.

## Frequently Asked Questions

**Question:** I have difficulty feeling the cool blood returning, although I can feel the pulsing. Any advice?

**Response:** As usual, the answer is "Practice Practice Practice!" The practitioner requires knowledge, depth, and detail to experience the sensations we're discussing. The knowledge part means you need to know your anatomy so that you can identify and feel all your pulses. In this meditation this includes the pulses of the axillary, brachial, radial, carotid, and temporal arteries, as well as the popliteal, femoral, iliac, and inferior vena cava veins. Know that the blood returns to the right side of the heart and exits via the left side to the systemic circulation. It is worthwhile learning the lower limb arteries, upper limb veins, the chambers of the heart, and the pulmonary circulation as well. These blood vessels are used in the next meditation, the Moment of Emptiness.

It is also important to know some of the traditional Chinese medicine physiology involved with this meditation. Understand that yang and hot energies rise. This is why people get migraines, insomnia, or plain old hot-headedness! Cold energies descend, which means patients get cold feet, lumbago (back pain), and some urinary symptoms.

Depth is required to improve the quality of your meditation. Quality can include two aspects: the first is the ability to use your mind's eye for detail, and the second is the ability to merge various senses and energies. Use the physical movement of rocking to help differentiate the arterial from the venous phases. Merging of the senses and being entranced by the pulse is part of the return to fetal consciousness. This comes with practice, simplification of your life, and the harmonization of your energies.

The Moment of Emptiness

1. Begin this meditation by tuning in to the pulsing of the heart and all major arteries. Check this against the actual pulse felt at your neck (carotid) or wrist (radial) arteries.

2. Become aware of the pause after arterial outflow. This is the first moment of emptiness that you should focus on. When first beginning this meditation, this moment is enough. Try to enlarge the moment of emptiness and consequently slow the pulse down. Merge the feelings of love and joy into this emptiness. Don't progress further until you have mastered steps 1 and 2.

3. Become aware of the venous return of blood to the heart.

4. Become aware of the pause after the venous return phase.

5. This is a second moment of emptiness before the heart contracts again. Focus on this period as well.

6. Merge these two periods or moments of emptiness into one.

7. If practicing this meditation in isolation, collect the energy in the lower tan tien and Turn the Wheel. Ideally this is done 360 times back to front and, then 360 times front to back.

## Commentary

**Goals and Advice:** The aim of this meditation is to find a moment of stillness amid the busyness of the heartbeat and its contractions. Finding stillness is paramount to realizing the One. The pulsing exercise above can be used initially to identify the two polarities, but after that, the student needs to dissolve this polarity.

There are two alternative meditations with this formula. One is more difficult than the other. The first—the simpler version—is to keep the body still and sense the outflow of blood as the period of activity. In between the periods of activity there is stillness. This is shown in fig. 6.2a, which is merely an arterial waveform tracing that is used in Western medicine. This is like a daily earth cycle where the night is still but the day is active.

The second version is to focus on two periods of stillness within a cardiac cycle. There is a moment of stillness after arterial contraction and another after the venous return phase. The way to feel this is to allow the body to rock forward and backward with each cardiac cycle. The forward and backward movements can be in a straight line or, even better, as part of a circle.

You can verify that the cycle is occurring once per heartbeat by feeling your carotid pulse during each cycle. You will notice that during arterial outflow the body rocks forward. During venous return the body rocks backward. Now there are two moments in each cardiac cycle when the body is vertical. These are the stillpoints to focus the mind on (fig. 6.2b).

If you can create a circle, then the center of the circle is the moment of emptiness. This is similar in some respect to the twice-a-year autumn and spring equinoxes. Creating a circle also means that this meditation can merge with the practice of spiraling. The Central Thrusting Channel is the stillpoint around which everything revolves—like the Pole Star.

Furthermore, you can create a sense of upper and lower poles of the body. This will focus the stillpoint within the heart in the Central Thrusting Channel. This stillpoint can then amplify until it fills the entire consciousness. This meditation is terrific, as it has a real sense of both time and space!

## Frequently Asked Questions

**Question:** This is really difficult, feeling the moment of stillness. Do you have any other hints?

**Response:** There are a couple of ways to access this stillness. Certainly do not use the monkey mind (horse intellect), but go deeper and return

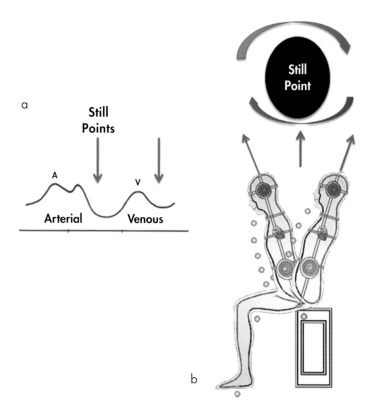

Fig. 6.2. Arterial and venous waveforms during a cardiac cycle:
the period of stillness corresponds to the center point when rocking.

to the infant mind. Think of yourself as a baby being nursed by your mother. Being held close to the heart and feeling loved and safe. Allow the heartbeats to become your lullaby as you enter a meditative state (not a sleep). Focus on those alternating stillpoints until they become more prominent. Don't worry too much if you can't sustain it for long periods. There will be benefits even if you don't achieve the goal of this exercise. The stillness and pulsing will open your channels and allow you to access a deeper state of consciousness! After a period of concentration, just allow yourself to move on to other formulas within the Greatest Kan and Li armamentarium.

Macrocosmic Meditation

The aim of this meditation is to expand your sense of self to include the entire visible universe. In essence, you become a cosmic being akin to a deity. According to traditional Taoism, the planets and stars should be ingested because they contain high levels of knowledge and wisdom. All material entities must be merged—from our organs, glands, and bones to the galactic material of the cosmos. In order to connect with the Wu Wei, you must first connect with everything. Once you have connected with everything, you proceed with the principles of coupling to reduce the multiplicity to a duality, and then the duality into One. The path from the material to the immaterial is then complete.

Within the Taoist framework, there are diverse variations on the Macrocosmic/Cosmic Being meditations. Three such formulas are given below.

## Macrocosmic Meditation: First Formula

This meditation is similar in principle to the Heavenly Stems and Earthly Branches formula, in that it also connects our body to the planetary bodies within our solar system. In this meditation, the heart becomes Mars, the liver Jupiter, the spleen Saturn, the kidneys Mercury, and the lungs Venus (fig. 6.3).

1. Connect the left hand to the liver, the right hand to the lungs, the left foot to the kidneys, and the right foot to the heart. Connect the spleen to the cauldron.
2. Next, connect Jupiter to the right parietal bone, liver, and left hand; Mars to the frontal bone, heart, and right foot; Saturn to the center of the crown, to the spleen, and the cauldron; Venus to the left parietal bone, lungs, and right hand; and Mercury to the occipital bone, kidneys, and left foot. Keep this order as it maintains the Creation Cycle, and don't forget to switch hands and feet if you are in the Southern Hemisphere.

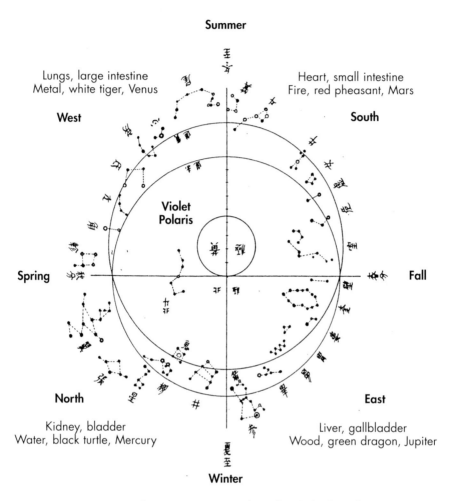

Fig. 6.3. Twenty-eight Lunar Mansions aligned with the four directions

The sun can occupy the left eye, although it can also replace the solar plexus or heart. The moon can become the right eye or the kidneys as well. The constellation projections can also vary. The first variation associates the center with Earth or Saturn. If you use the twenty-eight Lunar Mansions, then the four mythological creatures mark the four directions as follows: the Black Tortoise (left foot) is the north and is centered around the constellation of Aquarius; the Red Pheasant (right foot) is the south, centered around Leo; the Dragon (left hand) is east and centered around Scorpio; the White Tiger (right hand) is west and gathered around Aries. Note that the right and left are switched depending whether you are face up or down.

## 🜨 Macrocosmic Meditation: Second and Third Formulas

In the second formula, the head becomes the northern constellations while both feet become the southern constellations. The third formula puts Earth/Saturn at the center rather than the Pole Star. With these variations the reader will realize that the principle is more important than the details of the formula.

## Commentary

**Goals:** The planets, stars, and constellations represent missing aspects of our soul and spirit that must be integrated for us to progress. Each one is a profound symbol in and of itself, symbolic of a god and part of our quest for immortality. The principle is to connect and imagine yourself as large as the firmament: the details of which body part you connect with which heavenly bodies are of secondary importance.

**Advice:** My first piece of advice is to not get too pedantic over left hand versus right, as the confusion will impede your practice. Most important is that you imagine your body taking up the entire universe. One has to move from two-dimensional to three-dimensional awareness. Whether your left hand stays connected to the liver and right hand connected to the lungs depends on which direction you are facing. So you can do the opposite if you want to. However, remember that the kidneys will change north or south depending upon whether you are in the Northern or Southern Hemispheres. The cold (kidneys) is north in the Northern Hemisphere, while the cold direction is south in the Southern Hemisphere. Further advice for these meditations is similar to the suggestions for the Heavenly Stems and Earthly Branches practice: become familiar with the constellations around the poles and those that run along the ecliptic (fig. 6.4). For the Western student, the traditional twenty-eight Lunar Mansions may be quite difficult to learn; it may be helpful to start with the signs of the Western zodiac instead. Remember that the Lunar Mansions are basically the Western zodiac divided into smaller constellations to cover the twenty-eight day lunar cycle. Again, in this modern era, mobile-phone applications can assist you in locating the constellations you need. Alternately, you can obtain a planisphere from a bookshop or local observatory and calculate the whereabouts of the constellations by yourself.

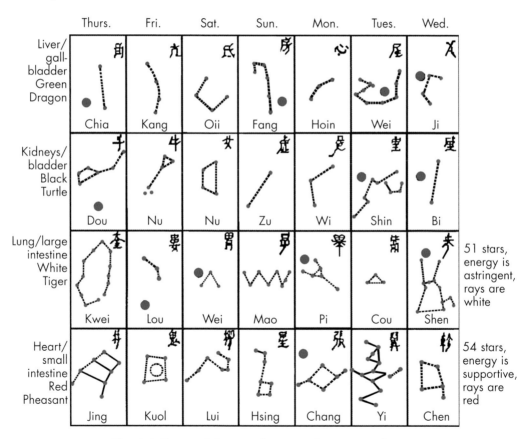

Fig. 6.4. Twenty-eight constellations with correspondences
to the four mythical creatures and solid organs in the second formula

Gathering the Lesser Medicine

The Lesser Medicine is a term used to describe the energy that results when the embryo merges with the Greater Spirit and facilitates complete merging of all the adept's inner spirits.

The Greater Spirit manifests as a powerful light or vortex and could be the Celestial Emperor or the Cinnabar Sovereign from the Three Pure Ones. The embryo has already been formed in Lesser Kan and Li. With the coupling in the heart tan tien, the coupling and orgasm reach a peak. The orgasm becomes very light and rises to the mid-eyebrow, where it not only attracts the Greater Spirit but also merges the Higher Shen from the brain with the other inner spirits.

1. After coupling and steaming for some time, you will begin to feel the essence in the cauldron as relatively pure. With this purity, consciousness has expanded such that the mind connects with deep outer space. The orgasm then becomes so pure and light that it rises to the mid-eyebrow.

2. At some point an inner light or vortex (often called the "first light") will appear in the middle of the universe. The light may be dim at first and look like a cloud. Gradually, however, the power of the Greater Spirit will activate all of your senses and emotional body.

3. The Higher Shen, manifesting as light and vibration in the brain, submits and joins with the Greater Spirit in a total reunification of all your inner spirits.

4. Bring the inner light and orgasm to the cauldron in the heart. Allow it to bathe in the heart tan tien's vapors and steam. You may condense the light by using the pakua.

5. Lower the light into the lower cauldron and condense it into a thick energy or pearl: this is the Lesser Medicine.

6. Move the Lesser Medicine in the Microcosmic Orbit (Turning the Wheel).

7. If practicing this meditation in isolation, collect the energy in the lower tan tien and Turn the Wheel. Ideally, this is done 360 times back to front and then 360 times front to back.

## Commentary

**Goals:** The goal of this meditation is to complete the process of reunification of the Nine Spirits through the invocation of the Greater Spirit. For the Westerner, the Greater Spirit is probably best understood in Christian terms: it is similar in principle to baptism by the Holy Spirit. Once all the fragmented spirits partake in this vision of the Greater Spirit, they voluntarily decide to work together as a team and merge into one. This includes the merging of the Higher Shen to complete the formation of the Supreme Commander (Yi-heart-mind power). The combined Higher Shen and fragmented shen can merge with the remainder of the Nine Spirits and form the Original Spirit (Yuan Shen). In Lesser Kan and Li we merged the Liver spirit (Hun). In Greater Kan and Li there was merging of the Thinking Spirit (Yi). The other spirits are joined in the journey from the lower tan tien to the crown along the Central Thrusting Channel. Now that the Higher Shen has returned, the process of becoming immortal is near complete.

**Advice:** At this stage of development of the embryo, there is not much to "do." The student needs to let go to the process. This means to continue coupling in the heart and stay in the moment. When the moment is right, the light of the Greater Spirit will appear. The ability to recognize the inner light is facilitated by dark room practice. The feelings and other senses awakened with this reunification signify its importance.

As we discussed earlier, the embryo is rarely sensed as an actual body with arms and legs. Rather, it is a deep sense of the primordial. To describe this state would be akin to verbalizing the Tao itself; it can really only be described in paradox and poetical form. There will be a sense of fullness yet emptiness. It is when there is light within darkness. It is where all echoes of the dragon and tiger can't be heard. It is full of vibration yet still. One's thoughts are paralyzed by its recognition.[1]

This realization of the embryo's indescribable nature is important, as students will want to grasp something tangible. Remember when the embryonic stage is complete it is no different from the accomplishments of other mystical traditions. It is equivalent to Enlightenment, achieving the wish-fulfilling gem, Nirvana, Christ Consciousness, or the philosopher's stone.

The recognition of the Greater Spirit is difficult to describe and is very personal. In meditation, many subtle lights and vortices can appear: the Greater Spirit will be the one surrounded by the most pleasant and beautiful experiences. In Taoist terminology this can be the energy of the Jade Emperor or the Cinnabar Sovereign. While these deities are anthropomorphized, they are in reality formless; hence we describe them as light or a vortex of energy.

In sum, the experience is a peak emotional and sensory one. Untold bliss, joy, peace, gratitude, and reverence are some of the many ways practitioners describe their experience. These feelings can be accompanied by blinding light, celestial music, fragrant flowers, or a dancing transparent vortex, among other possible sensory descriptions. Again, the story of Christ can aid the Westerners' understanding. When Jesus was baptized by John the Baptist, "the heavens were opened and he saw the Spirit of God descending like a dove and settling on him."[2]

##  Birth of the Spiritual Infant

With orgasm, the Great Spirit enters into the fetus as light, making it ready for birth and exiting the body. Lower abdominal movements indicate embryonic breathing (Womb Breathing) and the completion of the embryo's gestation. The adept's external breathing ceases and is replaced with the swallowing of chi. The embryo (Yuan Shen) is ready to rise and form the spiritual body, and thereafter partake in excursions through outer space and the Wu Wei (fig. 6.5).

This exercise begins when you have nurtured and carried the spiritual

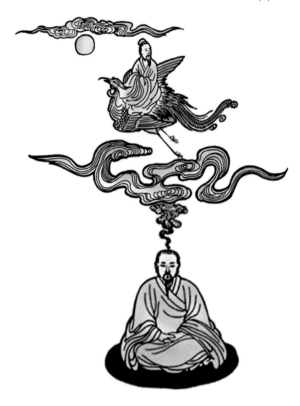

Fig. 6.5. The spiritual body, formed from the spiritual infant, has the ability to astral travel.

embryo in the lower tan tien for some time—traditionally ten months—called *lien hsu ho Tao*.[3]

1. When the embryo is ready you will see a powerful light outside of your body and coming from the heavens: this is the Greater Spirit. Mix this divine light with your embryo. The light may become wonderfully red—especially in the head—and you may hear heavenly sounds, perhaps including the merging of the dragon and tiger sounds (*Eeeeee* and *Ooommm*).

2. Seal all the senses tightly. Collect and swallow saliva; it will have a special fragrance and smell. The experience is akin to a divine orgasm. You should feel something move in the navel area. This bliss of all the senses can spread to involve the rest of the body, including the solar plexus cauldrons and the tip of the nose.

3. External breathing will have stopped at this point, and Womb Breathing will commence. This is the delicate inward and outer movement of the navel unaccompanied by external breath. The Womb Breathing is an indication that the embryo is ready for birth.

4. The embryo has now formed the Golden Elixir. Gestation is complete and the infant can now rise through the various cauldrons to form the spiritual body. Connection and travel through deep outer space and the Wu Wei can now occur.

5. If practicing this meditation in isolation, collect the energy in the lower tan tien and Turn the Wheel. Ideally this is done 360 times back to front, then 360 times front to back.

## Commentary

**Goals:** The goal now is to give life to the fully merged and developed embryo, which becomes an infant in the process. The infant can form a spiritual body and have an existence independent of your mortal body. This spiritual body can be used for space travel and ultimately for transformation of the physical to the spiritual; it is the vehicle for immortal ascension and the vehicle through which the dimensions of space, time, and observership can be united.

**Advice:** Giving birth to the inner child is also called the Great Medicine. In this advanced stage of Greatest Kan and Li, the spiritual fetus begins breathing on its own and is ready to be born. This is true internal breathing, and it results in the temporary cessation of the outer breath. At this point, the universal life force has entered your embryo, giving it the awareness and power of a baby god (also called the Red Baby). For those readers who understand the process of rebirth through Christian teachings, it is helpful to look to Jesus's exhortation that to enter the kingdom of heaven man must be born again. This formula teaches how the adept achieves this through meditation.

Nurturing the embryo through a full gestation is a process in itself, which may not be possible for adepts unable to go on a long retreat. Some texts literally advise ten months of continual practice on retreat to achieve this formula. Busy schedules interfere with gestation, and the adept may have to achieve repeated conceptions before a full-term fetus can be released.

Once the embryo is fully developed, the Golden Elixir (Yuan Shen) is achieved and immortality is inevitable. The Nine Spirits are unified! A state of spontaneity or "non-doing" exists. The embryo will naturally rise up without effort. Prior masters have equated this to ripened fruit naturally falling from a tree.[4]

Womb Breathing feels like an exaggerated but totally liberated cranio-sacral pump. It is more exaggerated as it involves the whole of the abdomen. Womb Breathing can gradually involve the entire body of the adept. It prepares the birth canal (the Central Thrusting Channel) for the release of the infant through the crown. Some adepts describe this birth as the flapping of the dragon's (or white crane's) wings. This movement accompanied by space travel is akin to immortal flight.

## Frequently Asked Questions

**Question:** Some of the older publications described three lights and mixing the light in the solar plexus cauldron rather than the heart caudron. Can you explain this?

**Response:** The process of giving birth to your embryo is shrouded in classical descriptions and current personal testimonies. The impregnation of the Great Spirit into your developed embryo is a profound event. The orgasm will involve all of your senses. The incoming inner light will be overwhelming. It is probably overly obsessive to say that you need to divide the process into three. The important point is that the light comes (first light), and your merged inner spirits also shine (second light), and then finally they merge into one (third light).

In regard to which cauldron—well, again, at that heightened level of meditation all cauldrons are firing and maybe even sensed as one. The focus of awareness can change from one to another. This is what Lu Dong-Pin and Chong Li-Chuan called the "stirring and tossing of the three tan-tiens."[5] So when the powerful light comes, just let go and see where the Great Spirit wants to fuse. In the resting phase, however, the fetus will return to the lower tan tien. When the infant wants to travel it must rise through the Central Thrusting Channel and through the crown. When it returns it can return to the lower tan tien.

**Question:** Can you explain the functions of the multiple cauldrons?

**Response:** In the Greatest Kan and Li we focus on the heart cauldron. The heart cauldron enables the embryo to be fed with the special energies and vapors of the heart. It offers the opportunity for the Shen to merge with the other spirits. The solar plexus offered an opportunity for the spleen spirit (Yi) to enter the embryo, while the lower tan tien offered an opportunity for the liver spirit (Hun) to seed it. The other spirits also merge with the embryo, but the exact timing of their joining the embryo is not as well defined.

The rising of the embryo through the various levels can also be seen as part of its education. Each level, including the upper tan tien and tip of the nose, offers a different environment and deep inner knowledge to the infant, so that it can be self-sufficient when it is born.[6]

**Question:** You equated the embryo stage with other religions. Do you think all religions are one?

**Response:** I (Andrew Jan) do believe that all the mystical religions share much common ground. I have briefly mentioned the accomplishments of Jesus and made comparisons to the Taoist system. These similarities include descriptions of the Wu Wei state of mind and concepts of rebirth and alchemy.

The question as to whether all religions have some core essence has been the subject of debate since the Age of Enlightenment, and has been supported by such authors/philosophers as William Blake (1788), William James (1902), Evelyn Underhill (1911), Aldous Huxley (1944), and Walter Stace (1960). These philosophers all supported the position that mystical experience is the central core of all religions, including Christian mysticism, Hinduism, Buddhism, and Sufism. In this light, the state of the Wu Wei is analagous with God and Emptiness; the embryo is equivalent to the philosopher's stone and the wish-fulfilling gem.

If the world would realize that all religions are one, then so much conflict could be avoided. It is in the rituals and dogma where differences lie; followers get attached to these rather than the core essence.

**Question:** Terms like "conception," "gestation," and "giving birth" seem fundamental to the practice. How real are they, or are they just metaphors to guide us?

**Response:** The immaterial worlds reflect the material world and vice versa; "as above so below."[7] Plato also outlined this principle in his Theory of Forms. Since creation and sexuality are the basic, fundamental laws of life and existence on this planet, how could they not also be reflected in the structure and forces of the immaterial world? I guess the problem is that the world of meditation seems so chaotic and ill defined. This makes everything difficult to grasp! I hope the formulas provide you with some assistance.

Cooking is the other foundation principle and metaphor that we use in Taoist alchemy. Cooking is the center of our lives and our homes. Why should it not be so in the meditation practices? Even if you're fasting, you still need to ingest and digest chi.

**Question:** These really are practices for prolonged retreat, aren't they?

**Response:** We will discuss this further in the final chapter of this book. However, keeping a pregnancy going long enough for the fetus to develop fully is a grand achievement. Living in a community has its stresses. These stresses can interrupt the pregnancy and often oblige the practitioner to begin the process over again. Getting sick will also cause a loss. The practitioner must guard and protect this process with absolute vigilance; in this sense, a prolonged period away with good support is ideal. The classics report ten lunar months, which corresponds to a normal physical gestational period. Perhaps this amount of time is necessary.

**Question:** Can you tell us about the stages after giving birth?

**Response:** After giving birth, the aim is to allow the spiritual body and the merged team of spirits to travel. Initially, consciousness can leave the body for a short time. Then later it can leave for prolonged periods of time.

According to Chang Po-Tuan, there is a breast-feeding stage that lasts for three years.[8]

The infant is nurtured for a long time until the future and past are understood. The next stage involves more prolonged periods of leaving the body. During these travels, space and all the universe's geography are condensed. After that is apparently a nine-year period of overwhelming emptiness and merging with the Wu Wei. The overwhelming nature of this stage feels like an insurmountable wall. However, after that, the sage reconnects to the beings of the world. The sage and all ordinary people become one!

Other facets of immortality can also be learned after the birth of the spiritual body. As discussed in chapter 2, actual physical ascension is an act of the spiritual body; in this case, the material is completely transformed to the immaterial. This level of accomplishment has been achieved by many Taoist masters, and occasionally by other adepts like Jesus of Nazareth.

Ending the Meditation:
Turning the Wheel of the Law

Each Kan and Li meditation should be ended with this formula, which is a process of collecting refined energy in the navel cauldron to be used in future meditations, including the higher levels. At this stage, the eyes are used to direct the energy produced by the meditation into the Microcosmic Orbit, guiding it into the cauldron behind the navel. This meditation is the same as used in Greater and Lesser Kan and Li Practices. We have reproduced the formula and accompanying text here.

1. Form a pool of sexual energy at the perineum. Looking straight ahead with your eyes closed, form a mental image of a clock with your eyes focused on its center.

2. Look down into the pool (6:00), and draw sexual energy up into the spine. The steam will travel up the spine drawing sexual energy with it (fig. 6.6).

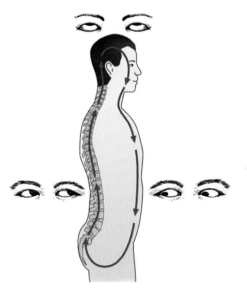

Fig. 6.6. Ending the meditation: Turning the Wheel of the Law

3. Look from the perineum up to the right (3:00 o'clock position with the clock facing forward, i.e., the coronal plane), drawing the energy up to T11 (in the sagittal plane), where it can be refined.

4. Look from the right up to the crown (12:00), and draw the energy there to further refine it at the pineal gland.

5. Look from the crown down to the left (9:00 o'clock in the coronal plane), and draw the energy down either through the tongue or through the thrusting routes into the cauldron at the navel. The energy is then stored in the cauldron.

   These four directions constitute 1 back-to-front round.

6. Repeat steps 1–5 above for at least 36 revolutions: you may do them in 4 rounds of 6 revolutions with 3 counts resting in between; or you may do 2 rounds of 12 revolutions with 6 counts of resting in between. In any sequence, the revolutions and resting counts must add up to 36. The rising steam will eventually flow independently of your counting, but maintain the mental revolutions to be sure the energy reaches the cauldron.

7. If you have time, do 4 rounds of 75 revolutions, resting for 15 counts in between rounds; or do 2 rounds of 150 revolutions, resting for 30 counts between rounds; or do 360 revolutions straight through. (All of these methods add up to 360, which is the maximum number of revolutions used to end this practice.) If you have less time, do 7 rounds, rest for 3 counts, then 15 rounds, rest for 3 counts, and finish with 7 more rounds. Practitioners should always finish with this as it helps gather any stagnant energy in the marginal aspects of the body. It also helps futher purify the energy experienced during the meditation and finally helps ground the adept prior to undertaking normal daily activities.

# Frequently Asked Questions

**Question:** Why is the turning of the Microcosmic Orbit at the end of the Kan and Li called the "Wheel of the Law?"

**Response:** The description of the Turning of the Wheel (Fa Lun) as a law was probably borrowed from the Buddhist tradition.[9] In order to find the way (or enlightenment), one had to follow laws like the Buddhist precepts and dogmas. Meditating on the Microcosmic Orbit was regarded as central to the dogma of concentration and mindlessness. In *The Secrets of the Golden Flower,* the Microcosmic Orbit (Turning the Wheel) became the central pathway to the Tao.

**Question:** What is the purpose of Turning the Wheel?

**Response:** According to Lu Dong-Pin, the Wheel maintains the blending and alchemical merging of the fragmented energies. This includes combining the five elements, refining yin and nurturing yang then finally fusing them, refining heaven and earth energies, circulating and merging blood and vapors, and forming the Original Spirit (Yuan Shen) from the five organ spirits.[10]

**Question:** How is the Wheel turned and how fast should it go?

**Response:** In the above meditation I usually encourage students to use their eyes or their mind only to Turn the Wheel. In *The Secrets of the Golden Flower* (Hui Ming Ching), Lu Dong-Pin suggests an alternative: Turning the Wheel in harmony with movement of the abdominal wall. Lu says, "Inhalation is accompanied by the sinking of the abdomen and exhalation by the lifting of it, but in these exercises the point is that we have a backward flowing movement as follows: when inhaling, one opens the lower energy gate and allows the energy to rise upward along the rear line of energy (in the spinal cord). . . . In exhaling, the upper gate is closed and the stream of energy is allowed to flow downward along the front line."[11]

Charles Luk bases his text on the teaching of Chao Pi-Chen, and claims that the setting up of the cauldrons and coupling creates an automatic spinning of the Wheel of the Law, which is accompanied by fetal or immortal breathing. Fetal breathing involves circulating the life force around the Microcosmic Orbit without external respiration. Immortal breathing includes the cosmos as part of one's body.

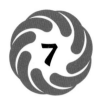

# Diet for the Greatest Kan and Li Practice

*When the five organs are rich and glossy the hundred channels are open and chi flows freely. When the hundred channels are open and chi flows freely the body fluids rise upwardly in proper accord. When the body fluids rise upward in proper accord, one does no longer think of the five flavors and will never be hungry or thirsty. One will expand one's years and ward off old age.*

HIGHEST CHI SCRIPTURE ON
NOURISHING LIFE AND EMBRYO RESPIRATION[1]

As Western practitioners, we can be inspired in our spiritual endeavors by the methods and achievements of the ancient Taoist adepts. It is a noble attribute to connect to the Taoist masters and immortals of old by reading the classics and practicing meditation. However, we should remember that using unproven outdated methods is fraught with risk. We are inspired by their supposed feats, yet this does not mean we should attempt to mimic them. As an ongoing principle, today's practitioners should seek current expert advice about modern safe methods. Students may still aim for high-level meditation experiences but without the risk of harm.

You, the reader, have a different body and mindset than the ancient Taoist adepts had, and consequently your practice should be less harsh. We will reiterate this point repeatedly in this chapter. Our purpose here is to inspire the reader to connect with the seemingly remarkable achievments of past masters. Furthermore, we can also be motivated to investigate some of their historical techniques. However, we do *not* advise readers to copy the herbal use and fasting techniques of the ancients. Most of the techniques, theories, and achievements recorded in the classics are both unproven and dangerous. Theories on the Three Worms are obviously outdated and would hold no credence in contemporary pathophysiology. TCM theories on the benefits of fasting also remain unsubstantiated. Practices were carried out by extraordinarily fit adepts within a supervising community who were readily willing to risk their lives. Specifically, the historical accounts of the miraculous health benefits of Kan and Li practice accompanied by fasting verge on the realm of myth and legend. At best, they serve as mere anecdotes of historical figures. Thus today, in the context of modern medicine, they would have little or no credence.

The risk of serious harm (not to mention death) for students is not acceptable in our modern society. Nevertheless, the Taoist retreat diet practiced at the Tao Garden under strict supervision, which includes partial fasting for a short finite period (maximum 19 days), is one practice that potentially supports and interacts with the specific practice of Kan and Li (fig. 7.1). This Pi Gu diet should never be practiced in isolation, nor without qualified supervision. Consultation and approval by your medical doctor before embarking on such a program is obligatory. If herbs are to be taken, it is imperative that you investigate these and consult a qualified herbalist for advice.

Much of this text is devoted to the premise that all the practices are a natural return to the Tao. When we orient ourselves to experiencing the primordial and the Wu Wei, perverse attachment and involvement

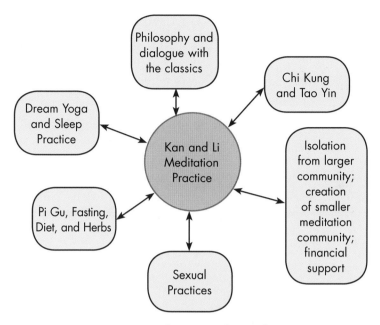

Fig. 7.1. Supporting the Kan and Li meditation practice

in worldly affairs naturally diminish. As we continue our journey toward the source, dietary change is inevitable. This is and should be a natural process as the student tidies up his or her diet with a gradual move toward balanced vegetarianism, support with safe herbs, gradual avoidance of grains, and short periods of partial fasting.

Kan and Li Practice lends itself to the retreat situation. Ideally, the student can arrange his timetable and affairs to have a break from everyday life and concentrate wholeheartedly on inner practice. The dietary and nutritional needs of adepts practicing intensive meditation on retreat are very different than those of practitioners who are involved in daily life. This chapter will focus deeply on several aspects of Taoist dietary practice during retreat, including the theory and practice of Pi Gu diets and fasting, Elixir Chi Kung practices, herbal supplements, and digestive health.*

---

*For more information about general UHT dietary guidelines, see Mantak Chia and William U. Wei, *Cosmic Nutrition* (Rochester, Vt.: Destiny Books, 2012).

## FACTORS AFFECTING DIET
## DURING KAN AND LI PRACTICE

Taoist adepts developed specific dietary guidelines in response to spiritual, physical, and environmental conditions. Physical isolation, limited physical activity, and the focus on returning to fetal physiology all contributed to the development of specific dietary practices (fig. 7.2).

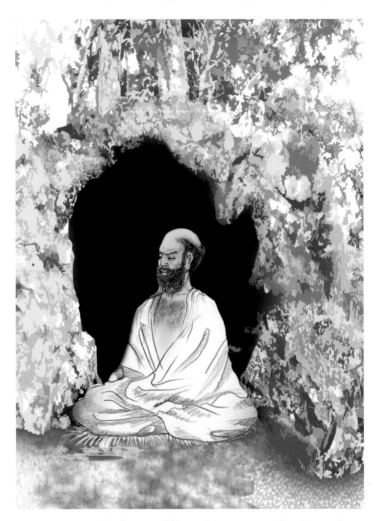

Fig. 7.2. Bodhidharma (fifth–sixth century CE) lived in and around a mountainous cave for nine years and practiced a form of Pi Gu.[2]

## Isolation with Change in Food Accessibility

Many adepts retreated to the mountaintops where access to food supplies from the towns was both difficult and expensive. In order to survive living at high altitude in the mountains, adepts had to learn to eat whatever plant material was available and nutritious. While this reasoning may not necessarily apply to the modern-day adept, who can organize medically qualified supervision and deliveries to the retreat setting, it is certainly true that the time usually devoted to earning an income so that food can be sourced, prepared, and digested is better utilized in meditation practice. In the immortal practices, this huge component of daily life is taken away.

## Returning to Fetal Physiology

*The individual returns to the primordial state of being and is like the embryo, but instead of being supported by a mother's body, he or she is nourished in the womb of the universe, the body corrected to be only Zhen Chi (True Chi).*

STEPHEN JACKOWICZ[3]

As we discussed in chapter 3, much of Taoist meditation theory relies on returning to and re-creating the fetal existence. In order to achieve fetal consciousness, the adept should mimic its dietary practices, breathing, light exposure, consciousness, and energetic patterns. In many respects this is what we do at the annual dark room retreats at Tao Garden in Chiang Mai, Thailand.

A fetus does not spend any time preparing meals or thinking about worldly problems. It merely floats in the dark womb sensing a pervasive love and connecting to the forces of life. The fetus does not eat, but continuously swallows amniotic fluid. The entire amount of amniotic fluid in a term fetus is 800 ml. Of this, the fetus swallows up to 94 percent of it at

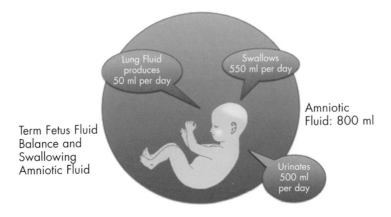

Term Fetus Fluid Balance and Swallowing Amniotic Fluid

Fig. 7.3. The fluid physiology of the fetus

an average of 500 ml per day (fig. 7.3). The practices of Elixir Chi Kung and ingestion of chi similarly nourish the adept in the fetal state. Note that urine contributes to the production of amniotic fluid.[4]

## Traditional Chinese Medicine Fasting Theory

In TCM theory, the normal state of being requires the energy of the spleen to govern digestion while the energy of the lungs extracts chi from the air. The purpose of digestion is to create energy. This energy is created from the combination of Food Chi and Air Chi together; this combination forms Gathering Chi, which combines with the Primordial Chi to form True Chi (Zhen Chi). True Chi has the functions of nourishing and defending the body. True Chi creates Ying Chi to nourish the internal organs and the rest of the body, and creates Wei Chi for immunity (fig. 7.4).[5]

As we approach the fasting state, we reduce the need for the lungs and spleen to expend their life force. We absorb Cosmic and Heavenly Chi directly from saliva and through the predominant energetic portals of the crown, third eye, and perineum. During fasting, it is air, chi, and saliva that produce the Gathering Chi; this combines with the Original Force to form True Chi (fig. 7.5). Therefore we enhance the mixing of saliva and

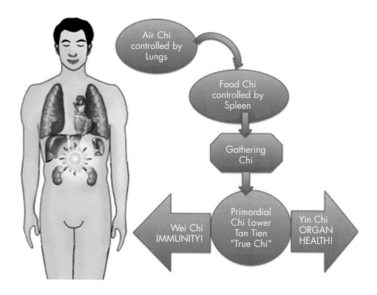

Fig. 7.4. Chi production in a nonfasting state

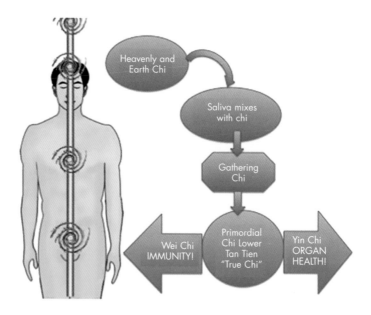

Fig. 7.5. The fasting state does not depend on
the spleen and lung for chi production.

Air Chi to encourage formation of Gathering Chi. Likewise we cultivate the Primordial Chi located in the lower tan tien so that the Gathering Chi can merge with the Primordial Chi to form True Chi and maintain immunity and organ health.

According to Kohn, fasting shuts down the lung and spleen and thereby creates a more primordial yin and yang exchange. The liver is soothed by isolation and the Tao Yin/Chi Kung practices. That leaves only the heart (yang) and the kidneys (yin) to interplay.[6] This model is consistent with the principles of Kan and Li practice wherein the five elements are reduced to a duality.

It is not difficult on an intensive meditation retreat to see how food interrupts one's meditation. When you spend one hour eating, you lose that time as well as additional time after eating, when your energy levels drop. This is likely to be the parasympathetic nervous system taking over, which is counterproductive to a prolonged meditation. After a postprandial nap, the channels block and one needs to start the meditation all over again. Conversely, meditation appears to appease hunger—like exercise—and to act as an appetite suppressant. Perhaps meditation produces hormones similar to those that signal satiety after eating.[7]

# PARASITE THEORY

## The Three Worms

As discussed in chapter 4, the Three Worms were likely to represent a combination of real worms (helminths) and blockages to the three tan tiens by spiritual beings that favored mortality rather than immortality.

In Traditional Taoist theory the Three Worms correlate with the three tan tiens. They can cause disease in both physical and psychoenergetic dimensions. A generalization of the disorders caused by the Three Worms includes the following: a worm in the upper tan tien (Peng Ju) causes excessive attachment to the senses. A worm in the heart (Peng Zhi) causes a background imbalance and negative emotional

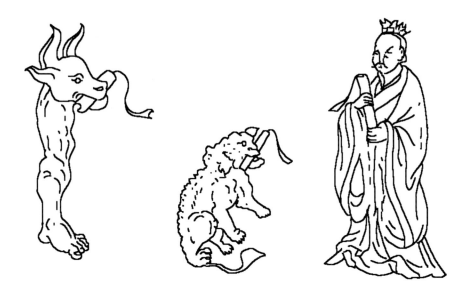

Fig. 7.6. The three malevolent worms:
Peng Ju, Peng Zhi, and Peng Jiaou

state, while a worm in the lower tan tien (Peng Jiaou) causes excessive lust and addictions (fig. 7.6).

Early Taoists thought that grains would nourish the Three Worms while fasting, while certain herbs and practicing Chi Kung would eliminate them. Elixir Chi Kung in particular was oriented to the expulsion of the Three Worms (*san shi*). The third century CE treatise entitled *Imbibing the Five Chis* (Taishang Lingbao Wu Fu Xu) contains recipes for expelling the Three Worms that include eating asparagus and poke root and avoiding the five grains. "Thereupon begin to eat them while observing ritual prohibitions. In five days your food intake will start to decrease. After twenty days grains will be eliminated and your intestines will be so fat that they can only hold air. The various worms will all leave. Your ears and eyes will hear and see clearly. All of your moles and scars will disappear."[8]

Another prescription by the famous physician Hua Tuo (140–208 CE) states: "To expel the Three Worms, use a green pasty powder made from the leaves of the lacquer tree. Take it for a long time, and the Three Worms will be expelled, the five inner organs will be greatly strengthened. The body as a whole will feel light, and there will be no white hair."[9] It is now known that the leaves mentioned by Hua Tuo (*Toxicodendron vernicifluum*) contain the antioxidants butein and sulfuretin, and are still used in traditional Chinese medicine for the treatment of intestinal parasites. However, this is not substantiated by good current research with patient-oriented outcomes. It is known that this herb can cause significant adverse effects, such as dermatitis.

The Three Worms are intimately linked with health, longevity, and immortality. Remember the worms are also known as the Death Bringers. They block the life force to the three tan tiens. However, there is the concept of self-will here: there are Taoist writings that comment that an individual's choice determines whether the Death Bringers stay or go. They stay when the adept ultimately chooses death rather than immortality.[10]

## Western Parasite Theory

In Western biology, organisms that live in the gut can be positive (mutualists), neutral (commensals), or harmful (parasites). Man has always lived in harmony with the friendly bacteria and yeasts. They help create homeostasis within the intestine, maintaining correct pH levels, producing vitamins, and assisting with the digestion of food. The classic examples of friendly bacteria include *Bacteroides, Clostridium, E. coli, Lactobacillus, Peptococcus, Bifidobacterium, Fusobacterium, Eubacterium,* and *Ruminococcus.* Friendly fungi and yeasts include: *Candida, Saccharomyces, Aspergillus,* and *Penicillium.* However, there are apparently no friendly worms.

### *Do Parasites Create Disease or Does Disease Encourage Parasite Growth?*

Controversy exists as to whether organ imbalance results in overgrowth of parasites or whether the parasites themselves are the cause of organ imbalances. In the Western world where water and food supplies are essentially clean, the overgrowth of atypical parasites is likely to be a result (according to TCM and naturopathic theories) of imbalance of emotions, pathogenic factors, or other excesses that result in disease (fig. 7.7). This is opposed to the setting of ancient rural China where gross tapeworm, hookworm, and roundworm infections were common and significant.

In Western medicine today, diagnosis and treatment of worm infections is important mostly in regard to travelers, children, and those with immune deficiencies. In naturopathic medicine and TCM, chronic diseases are often thought to have a parasitic etiology.

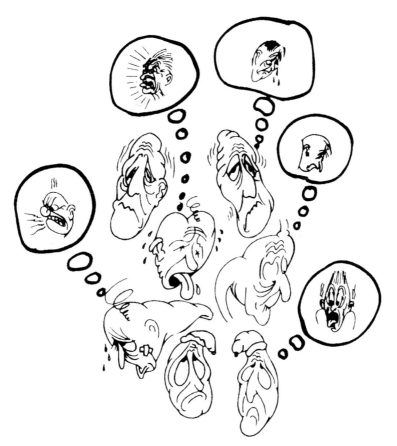

Fig. 7.7. Organ disease can arise from parasite
invasion or from unbalanced emotions. Organ disease can
also lead to parasite invasion.

### Western Methods of Eliminating Parasites

Parasite infections that have been medically diagnosed are usually treated with antiparasitic medications. In natural medicine practices, parasites are generally treated with dietary modifications, pre- and probiotics, and herbs. Antiparasitic diets vary but predominantly center on avoiding refined foods including grains and sugars. One should avoid coffee and alcohol. The efficacy of probiotics and prebiotics is unclear. However, ongoing research will make their clinical use clearer.

The World Gastroenterology Organization defines probiotics as: "Live microorganisms which, when administered in adequate amounts, confer a health benefit on the host (figs. 7.8 and 7.9)." Probiotics include: *Lactobacillus* bacteria, the yeast *Saccharomyces cerevisiae,* and some *E. coli.* Prebiotics, on the other hand, are nondigestible substances that provide a beneficial physiological effect for the host by selectively stimulating the favorable growth or activity of a limited number of indigenous bacteria.[11] Probiotics for the eradication of low-grade parasite infections in the Western population is not proven. There are, however, animal studies showing some favorable results with both probiotics and prebiotics.[12]

Probiotics have shown some efficacy in gastroenterological diseases including *H. pylori* infection, lactose intolerance, irritable bowel syndrome, antibiotic associated diarrhea, and enteritis in children.[13]

Traditionally foodstuffs such as garlic, pumpkin or papaya seeds, pomegranates, beets, and carrots were used to rid helminth infections naturally. Evidence for use of natural foodstuffs is substantiated only by small trials and therefore requires further research.[14]

## EMPTYING THE COLON

Emptying the colon via purgative herbs or colonic irrigation has become a common support practice for high-level meditation. There is a paucity of evidence to support these practices, although they are recommended

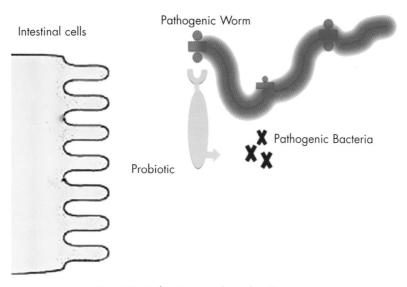

Intestinal cells

Pathogenic Worm

Probiotic

Pathogenic Bacteria

Fig. 7.8. Probiotics may have binding sites
that neutralize worms and pathogenic bacteria.

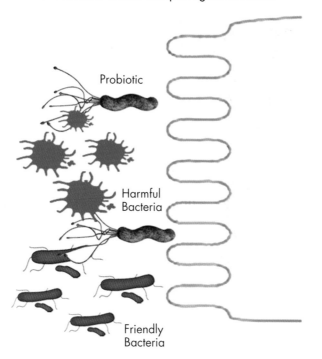

Probiotic

Harmful
Bacteria

Friendly
Bacteria

Fig. 7.9. Probiotic substances encourage the growth of
healthy bacteria and discourage harmful ones.

by expert opinion, anecdotal reports, and historical traditional usage.

In a recent publication on high-level yogic meditation, Swami Adiswarananda says, "Five things are indispensable for success in meditation: the practice of silence, a light diet of milk and fruits, living in solitude, personal contact with the teacher, and a cool place. Concentration and meditation should be practiced with an empty stomach, an empty bladder, and empty colon, and a salt free diet is immensely helpful in that regard."[15]

Traditionally, Taoists would use cathartic diets with herbs to empty the colon.[16] The physician Chang Tsung-Cheng states: "All physicians know that the unobstructed circulation of fresh blood and vital energy are the most important factors in health. But, if the stomach and bowels are blocked, then blood and energy stagnate."[17] It is common for practitioners entering the dark room and carrying out Kan and Li practice to reduce fecal loading by the use of gentle laxatives or having a colonic prior to entering (fig. 7.10). This gives a sensation of being light and empty. Furthermore, a bowel that is full of fecal matter can obstruct the energy that needs to fill the tan tien and abdomen during high-level practice.

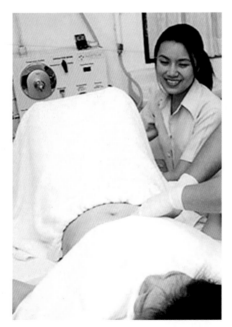

Fig. 7.10. Colonic therapy

The orthodox medical position is to "Advise patients that colon cleansing has no proven benefits and many adverse effects. Current evidence is inconsistent or of limited quality."[18] There have been no significant randomized trials of colonic therapy. Proponents of it argue vested interest and remind us that the overall complication rates of allopathic health care are higher than the complication rates from colonic irrigation. Nevertheless, the allopathic position should remind the student to investigate any colonic establishment before undergoing therapy. Understand that certain preparations can cause fluid and electrolyte imbalances, and that infections can result from inadequate maintenance or sterilization techniques. Bowel perforation can occur with excessive water pressures. Therefore cautious students wishing to empty their colon prior to high-level practice may go with safer techniques such as the use of gentle laxatives.

## ELIXIR CHI KUNG

*Rinsing and swallowing the Numinous Fluid (saliva)*
*puts a man beyond reach of the calamities.*
HUANG TING JING[19]

Elixir Chi Kung is an adjunct to Kan and Li Practice. It can be used as a warm-up (as discussed in chapter 4) or as part of the Kan and Li practice proper. Elixir Chi Kung can go by other names including "meals of emptiness" (Kung Fan)[20] and "saliva practice."

Swallowing saliva is a totally automatic practice that occurs in the blissful state of meditation when respiration nearly ceases. This is likely to be a fetal reflex, whereby in the womb the fetus survives on lower arterial oxygen saturations. It is difficult to separate swallowing saliva, high-level meditation (activation of the empty force, coupling, and absorbing essence), and fetal breathing. To pull these techniques apart is a useful exercise for teaching and learning, however, they are all ultimately joined in the same process of returning to the primordial.

From a Western viewpoint, saliva contains electrolytes, proteins, and hormones. Glucose is also excreted into the saliva. The electrolytes (sodium, potassium, bicarbonate, and chloride) are vital constituents of intra- and extracellular fluid. The proteins in saliva serve a variety of functions: amylase catalyzes the digestion of carbohydrates, lipase digests fats, B12 binding compounds aid in the absorption of vitamin B12, gustin assists taste perception, lysozyme is an antibacterial agent, glycoproteins act as lubricants. Additional proteins bind to tannins and other toxins in foodstuffs, so that they can move safely through the digestive system. Hormones appear in the saliva; it is controversial whether they accurately reflect the levels of hormones present in blood or tissue.

The average amount of saliva swallowed in a nonmeditational state is approximately 1.5 liters per day. This may be increased in high-level meditation practice, which might thereby increase the digestive, detoxificative, and immune functions of the practitioner. A foundation principle in Chi Kung is that "wherever the mind goes the chi will follow."[21] If you imagine or massage your endocrine glands, for example, while mixing and swallowing saliva, this has the potential to increase hormone levels in your saliva.

There has been no research on the specific effects of Elixir (Saliva) Chi Kung, although there are research papers showing that Chi Kung in general increases the amount of saliva[22] and its lysozymes.[23] The other part of Elixir Chi Kung is that the saliva combines with chi from the heavens, cosmos, and the earth. This elixir is then swallowed and combined with the original force to create True Chi. The absorption and filling of the tan tiens with chi may be the centerpiece of the healing process (fig. 7.11).

There is some discussion in *Golden Elixir Chi Kung* of oxygen mixing with the saliva.* From a Western medical viewpoint this doesn't make

---

*See Mantak Chia, *Golden Elixir Chi Kung* (Rochester, Vt.: Destiny Books, 2005).

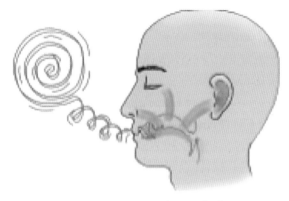

Fig. 7.11. Mixing saliva with chi

sense. Certainly the amount of oxygen required to maintain aerobic metabolism could in no way be met by this mode of absorption. What I (Andrew Jan) believe is that in the high-level meditation trance state, the swallowing reflex gets activated and respiration becomes so subtle as to remain undetected; this gives the perception that oxygen is being absorbed from saliva.

## Traditional Practices of Elixir Chi Kung

The practice of Elixir Chi Kung has a long history in Taoism. The following classics discuss Elixir Chi Kung, Pi Gu, and fasting practices, and as well as expelling the Three Worms.

> *Abstaining from Cereals and Consuming Qi* (Quegu Shiqi) (168 BCE)[24]
> *Supreme Purity Qi Regulation Classic* (Taiqing Tiaoqi Jing) (Tang dynasty)[25]
> *Scripture of the Yellow Court* (Huang Ting Jing) (Jin dynasty 265–317)[26]
> *Restoring the Primary Vitalities* (Hsi Yo Tou Hsien-Seng Hsui Chui Nan) (thirteenth century)[27]

*Imbibing the Five Chis* (Taishang Lingbao Wu Fu Xu)
   (Third century)[28]
*The Records of the Three Kingdoms* (San Guo Zhi)
   (Han dynasty)[29]
*How Immortals Give up Grain and Eat Qi* (Shen Xian Que
   Gu Shi Qi) (Han dynasty)[30]
*Greater Clarity Scripture on Balancing Chi* (Taiqing Tiaoqi
   Jing) (Tang dynasty)[31]
*Taiqing Zhong Huang Zhen Jing Scripture of the Realm of
   Grand Purity of the Central Yellow* (Fourth century)[32]
*The Scripture of the Foundation of the Tao on Expelling and
   Taking In* (Daojia Tuna Jing) (Seventh century)
Laozi Zhong Jing Central Scripture of Laozi (Third century)[33]

In the *Supreme Purity Qi Regulation Classic,* the practice involved rinsing and mixing saliva in the mouth, blocking loss of chi through the palms and soles, quieting and ceasing the breath, and swallowing warm chi to the heart and lower tan tien. This was to involve a few hundred swallowings per day.

The *Scripture of the Yellow Court* emphasized that longevity and cultivation of the spirit lies in nourishing the root of the spirit with saliva. The root of the spirit is the lower tan tien. Chapter 3 of this treatise tells us that "Rinsing and swallowing the spirit fluid (saliva) can prevent all kinds of diseases, wash away dirty things inside of the body, and make our bodies look magnificent with shining skins and smell like orchids and have a healthy complexion."[34]

This Elixir Chi Kung practice from the Northern Sung dynasty was said to rid the body of the Three Worms.

The Jade Spring water is the secretion of the two vessels underneath the tongue. Every morning sit up, close your eyes, clear your mind of all anxiety, gnash the teeth 27 times until the mouth is full, then rinse the teeth with it and swallow it, keeping in mind that you are sending it (to the lower region of vital heat) below the umbilicus, through the Pool of Chi. For some time it makes a noise like a waterfall flowing deep in a grotto. In this way the circulation in all the vessels and tracts is harmonized.[35]

In the thirteenth century, a teacher named Tou listed the important components for rejuvenation: Tuo (saliva), Hseuh (blood), Mo (vessels and nerves), Chi, Shui (juice of organs), Ching, and Shen.[36]

> *I supped the Six Chi; drank the Night Dew.*
> *Rinsed my mouth in the Sun Mist; savoured the Morning*
>     *Brightness*
> *Conserving the pure fluid of the spiritual light.*[37]

In this poem (by an unknown author written approximately 110 BCE), the "night dew" is the saliva and the "chi" would be the combined essence of the sun, the morning freshness, and the inner light (fig. 7.12).

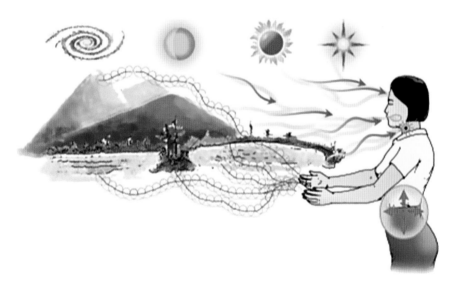

Fig. 7.12. Saliva combines with chi from
the heavens, cosmos, and the earth.

# Modern Elixir
# Chi Kung Practices

In Mantak Chia's *Golden Elixir Chi Kung,* there are over eight different formulas to practice.* One of these practices is Shaking the Head and Wagging the Tail, included below.

 ## Shaking the Head and Wagging the Tail

1. Stand with the legs shoulder-width apart.
2. Perform the next four movements simultaneously, for a total of about 2 minutes.
   a. Extend your arms straight out in front of the chest. Make thundering palms by rubbing the palms together back and forth against each other to generate the heat.
   b. Shake the head to the right and left.
   c. Wag your pelvis and sacrum in the opposite direction of the head. Act like you are wagging a tail attached to the coccyx.
   d. Draw your sense organs into the head. Collect and beat the saliva in your mouth until it is very thick.
3. Use the heat in the palms to cover both temples. Move the thundering palms to cover the solar plexus, which corresponds to the hours of 11 p.m.–1 a.m., the Gall Bladder meridian hour.
4. Feel the point radiate with increasing chi. Circulate the chi and blood into the gallbladder.
5. Gather the chi from the hair all around the body. Suck saliva into the mouth and mix it with the Universal Chi.
6. Swallow the saliva into the solar plexus and feel the saliva turn into chi at this hour/point. Feel your hands become warm.

---

*See Mantak Chia, *Golden Elixir Chi Kung* (Rochester, Vt.: Destiny Books, 2005).

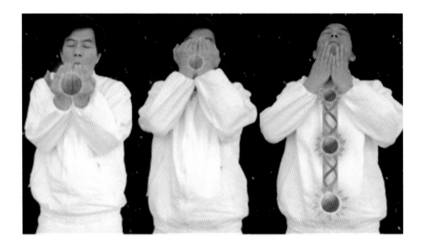

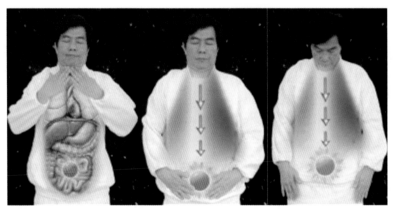

Fig. 7.13. Elixir Chi Kung: swallowing the chi

7. Repeat steps 3–6 for the following the points:
   a. Chi Chung (navel) (5–7 p.m.): Rub hands hot and cover the navel, swallowing the saliva to this point (fig. 7.13).
   b. Yin Tang (third eye) (7–9 a.m.): Rub hands hot and cover the third eye, then swallow the saliva to this point.
   c. Jade Pillow (Base of skull—GV 16) (9–11 a.m.): Rub hands hot and cover the point, then sallow the saliva to this point.
   d. Da Zhui (GV 14—back base of the neck) (3–5 a.m.): Rub the hands hot and cover the point, then swallow saliva to this point.
   e. Ming Men (GV 4—lower back) (1–3 p.m.): Rub hands hot and

cover the Ming Men point at Lumbars 2 and 3. Swallow the saliva to this point.

f. Chang Qiang (GV 1—coccyx) (3–5 p.m.): Rub hands hot and cover the sacrum, letting the tip of your finger touch the coccyx; swallow saliva to this point.

8. Collect energy at navel to complete the practice.

## PI GU DIET AND FASTING

*Pi Gu* literally means to "avoid grains," and classically refers to these five: glutinous millet, panicled millet, rice, soybeans, and wheat.[38] Of course, soybean is not a grain but a legume, but the ancients may not have had such a formal classification of foodstuffs. Other grains include: oats, sorghum, rye, and buckwheat. For developing countries the grains constitute a large portion of the diet; this is less so in developed nations.

Avoiding grains has traditionally been considered a transition diet to becoming a complete breatharian, or one who eats chi.* The classical term for fasting is *Bu Shi,* "not eating." Pi Gu can consist of partial or complete fasting. Partial fasting would focus on the avoidance of grains. According to David Palmer: "Partial fasting involved taking only small quantities of water, fruits, or other foods."[39] Another variation of Pi Gu is a stone diet used by the External Alchemists, as mentioned in chapter 1. The transition diet should be carried out under appropriate supervision such as is offered at the Tao Garden. The authors do not recommend complete or partial fasting without consultation with a suitably experienced and qualified health practitioner. Partial or complete fasting also requires constant supervision. In the Tao Garden Darkness Kan and Li retreat, participants touch base with instructors several times a day. Any untoward symptoms

---

*Some authors, such as Eskilden, argue that Pi Gu actually means not eating any food.[40] He bases this in part on the tendency of Chinese language and culture to describe general aspects of food as grains. He cites the example of *chifan,* which literally translates as "eating rice" but means "to eat."

are acted upon. Medical care can be accessed easily. Often simple actions such as an increase in food intake are instigated. Withdrawal from the partial fasting program is encouraged where indicated. The student is reminded that the meditation experiences are the goal, not the forced starvation of the body.

The purpose of the Pi Gu diet from a TCM perspective is to reduce the burden on the spleen, so that its energy can be used in other ways. This redirection of energy is noticed as the disappearance of postprandial (postmeal) symptoms like sleepiness and an inability to meditate. As stated above, saliva gathers the chi, which is then taken down to the lower tan tien to form True Chi, which nourishes the blood and organs. Chi can also directly be gathered into the lower tan tien from the energetic portals of the Bahui, Yintang, Laogung, Yongquan, and Huiyin (crown, third eye, palms, soles, and perineum).

For those adepts who have not built up their Chi Kung to the stage of fasting, TCM principles indicate that the vital organs require vital substrates to tonify and replenish. In the aging kidneys, chi and yin are gradually lost so foodstuffs must be chosen to support these functions. Foods that moisten and soften the liver and heart are also helpful, while foods that overstress or dampen the spleen must be avoided. Please note, however, that all individuals will have different constitutions from a five-element perspective, and thus different strengths and weaknesses. Therefore the diet will have to be modified according to the individual adept.

From a Western perspective, the following dietary components are fundamental: amino acids to repair proteins; nucleic acids to repair DNA and RNA; vitamins to assist with vital chemical pathways that act as coenzymes and catalysts; minerals to act as important chemical substrates for body fluids, cellular excitation, and nutritional transport and metabolism, and alternative energy sources to carbohydrates and animal fats.

## Pi Gu as a Transition to Fasting

Dated information on the ancient practicalities of Pi Gu as a transition diet can be obtained from the classics. The first documented Taoist book of fasting is suitably titled *Giving Up Grain and Eating Chi* (Quegu Shiqi); it dates approximately from 168 BCE and was found with the discovery of the Mawangdui tombs.[41]

Another important text is *The Greater Clarity Scripture on Balancing Chi* (Taiqing Tiaoqi Jing), from the Tang dynasty.[42] This text provides Chi Kung, supplementary Saliva Chi Kung, meditation exercises, and information about living according to the chi cycle.* Specific advice includes: Do not force the avoidance of grains; this should happen naturally. If you find yourself forcing, you will get sick. For the early transition phases, the book advises small unflavored amounts of cooked oats and rice, and the avoidance of raw food, roots, and old and greasy foods.

Go Hung reminds us that "One has to train for this beforehand and not make an abrupt break from cereals."[43] In the *Bao Pu Tzu* he recommended a diet of pine nuts and roots (burdock). Go Hung also comments that Taoists wandering the mountains would live on small amounts of dried meat and alcohol.[44] Schipper points out that as soon as a Taoist practitioner requires grains, he ends up becoming a part of the agricultural community. Because grains were a phenomena deeply intertwined with life, giving them up was a way of avoiding mainstream society, not just avoiding cereals specifically.

*How Immortals Give Up Grain and Eat Chi* (Shenxian Quegu Shiqi) advises the ingestion of potentially toxic actractylis cakes, dates, saliva, and water to ward off severe hunger:

> If after two or three days of this your stomach feels irritated and has a
> strong sensation of hunger, take nine ripe dates or nine square atractylis

---

*For information about living according to the chi cycle, see *The Practice of Greater Kan and Li,* chapter 8.

cakes and eat them one at a time morning and evening. Do not take any more food than that. Really if you do not think about food you will find no need to eat. As for drinking water, you take three or five pints every day spaced out evenly. Do not stop drinking. Also it is a good idea to keep a date pit in your mouth. It enhances the chi in your body and provides a steady flow of saliva.[45]

The dark room retreats at Tao Garden rely on a Pi Gu diet that avoids cereals while maintaining essential foodstuffs for the novice embarking on this path. This diet is continually being refined and readers are advised to attend the Tao Garden dark room retreats for information on current safe practice. Below is a sample menu from a 2011 dark room retreat.

> *Breakfast:* egg white, cooked peanuts (2 to 3 handfuls), and an apple
>
> *Lunch:* sesame or vegetable broth soup, green soybeans (2 handfuls in pods), watermelon (5 pieces), and honey sesame biscuits
>
> *Dinner:* cooked pumpkin (1 piece), raw tomatoes, and a pear
>
> *Herbal teas taken during day:* a variety of teas including choices from burdock, turkey rhubarb, sheep sorell, slippery elm, cress, senna leaf, buckthorn, peppermint leaf, uva ursi leaf, orange peel, rose hip, marshmallow, honeysuckle, and chamomile
>
> *Chinese herbs:* twice per day

This diet eliminates the cereal grains, but it does not exclude the soybean. With more advanced training, soy could be excluded as well. The amounts are small but adequate to sustain the novice for several weeks given prior good health and participation in an effective meditation and Chi Kung schedule.

### *TCM Comments*

From a traditional Chinese medicine perspective, peanuts are warming. They are slightly sweet, hence in small amounts they positively affect the spleen. (In Western society peanuts are often served with salt, which can drain kidney yin and Jing, but salt is not included in the dark room diet.) Egg white is cooling and helps with sleeping. Pumpkin is also cooling and has a sweet and bitter taste. In small amounts, this sweet/bitter combination supports the spleen. The bitter flavor also affects the small intestine and has some antihelminthic (worm-destroying) properties.

Like most fruits, apples are cooling. They are both sweet and sour and hence affect the spleen and liver. With their malic and tartaric acids, apples are good for indigestion. The pectin found in apples can apparently chelate heavy metals and also has a positive effect on lowering cholesterol.[46]

Watermelon is very cooling and hence ideal for Kan and Li practice, which can produce a lot of heat leading to dehydration and constipation. Watermelon's sweet flavor benefits the spleen and digestion. The seeds have positive nutritional value and can be ingested in small amounts. Because they are black and almost kidney shaped, the seeds support the kidneys. Watermelon seeds contain cucurbocitrin, which has a vasodilatory effect and can lower blood pressure; it should be ingested with caution.[47]

The description, potential benefits, and harms of the herbs and herbal teas listed above are beyond the scope of this text. The reader is encouraged to investigate these herbs according to the principles cited at the end of the chapter before consumption, and before attendance at the Tao Garden Darkness Kan and Li retreat.

 ## Practice for a Pi Gu Diet

The act of eating is performed as a modified Elixir Chi Kung practice.

1. Sit comfortably.

2. Bless your food.

3. Smell the food.

4. Identify the food, then visualize its origin and growth, thereby connecting to the sun, seasons, water, nitrogen sources, etc.

5. Taste the food and chew it until it becomes liquid. Really work the saliva.

6. Feel the food influenced by the spleen and stomach becoming Food Chi (Gu Chi). Sense the air under the influence of the lungs becoming Air Chi (Kong Chi).

7. Combine Air, Earth, Cosmic, and Heavenly Chi with your saliva and the emulsified food. Together they become Gathering Chi.

8. Collect the Gathering Chi in the lower tan tien. Under the influence of the kidneys, the Gathering Chi combines with the primordial force to become True Chi. Feel the kidneys and the primordial force combining with the Gathered Chi.

9. True Chi nourishes the organs (Ying Chi) and provides immunity (Wei Chi). Feel the organs shiny and radiant. Feel an aura of protection around you (fig. 7.14).

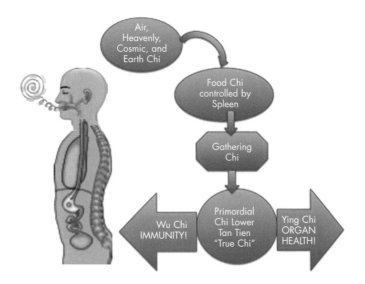

Fig. 7.14. Pi Gu practice

# Pi Gu Teachings from the Classics

Several of the classics address the specific needs and practices associated with fasting, and with the transition to fasting.

### *Zhong Huan Jing*[48]

The Zhong Huan Jing is an ancient classic that suggests swallowing air as the mainstay of fasting. Its strict regime begins with the immediate cessation of solids. Practice begins with lying down at midnight. The adept goes into meditation, swallowing air and commencing fetal respiration. This practice is used to ward off hunger. Although discouraged from drinking fluids, the adept is allowed herbal teas and soups. The text recommends sesame seed soup and powdered tuckahoe (Fu Ling)[49] mixed with small amounts of milk and honey. Apparently they act as an appetite suppressant and diuretic. The text warns the adept about the significant side effects of these herbs and practices.

There is an overtone in the Zhong Huan Jing text that implies that the techniques are forced and require strenuous discipline. Furthermore, these forced techniques are likely to be dangerous. In the UHT dark room practice in Chiang Mai we teach the opposite: that this fasting and swallowing is an effortless manifestation of getting into a deep meditative state. When one couples, the swallowing reflex activates, respiration almost ceases (Fetal Breathing), and the appetite is suppressed naturally. The secret is not the monkey-mind activation of swallowing air but staying in a trance state or deep meditation state that wards off hunger and activates the spontaneous swallowing of saliva and air. The quaternary of deep coupling, fetal breathing, air swallowing, and fasting become inseparable in high-level meditation states. This is why so many of these classics talk about eating chi and swallowing air. The impressive mind and health claims, as well as the duration of fasting reported in the Zhong Huan Jing and other ancient texts cited below, are unsubstantiated. While not intending to degrade the supernatural achievements and duration of fasting achieved by adepts in these texts, the reader is reminded that such feats belong to "superheroes" or "immortals" in the realm of myth and legend. Their reported practices are of historical and legendary interest but are not to be used as a guide for modern-day practice.

With progress in meditation and withdrawal from solid food, fecal matter is reduced. With further practice the lower, middle, and upper tan tiens fill with chi. Alongside these changes, the body becomes healthy and the mind achieves clarity. The Zhong Huan Jing text predicts the following time sequence: one month for the lower tan tien to fill; two months for the middle tan tien, and three months for the upper tan tien to open. At this hundred-day mark the mind is lucid and clear and the organs are sensed as bright and lubricated. At the three-hundred-day mark the adept fends off demons and ghosts, and immortal status is achieved after a thousand days.

The second chapter of the Zhong Huan Jing attempts to reassure the adept that the side effects of weakness, loss of weight, and the pale-yellow pallor are transitory. It provides commentary on the ridding of the psychophysical Three Worms and their natures. As discussed earlier, the Three Worms are intermingled with the adept's attachment to the material plane: they will overwhelm the adept with mood swings and cravings for luxuries, sex, food, and social contact. However, once the Three Worms have been conquered, the mind becomes clear.

The third chapter of the Zhong Huan Jing highlights the positive end-state, which includes the permanent opening of the tan tiens and clarity of mind with the removal of all falsehoods. One becomes like a god and lives in a conscious state filled with deities. One reaches the immortal realm.

There is a positive twist to the initial withdrawal and isolation from the community: the treatise claims that the adept's organs become so positive and healthy that they now possess divine powers. The heart and liver have the power to cure human disease. Lung Chi is used for reading minds and fortune telling. Spleen Chi enables the student to dematerialize and manifest as an apparition in order to inspire lay persons and adepts to embark on their spiritual journeys. Thus the successful adept now returns to the community as a healer and forms a definitive relationship with her people.

The final chapters of the Zhong Huan Jing expand on how the adept can merge the Three Pure Ones and the body's spirits and engage in ongoing astral flight. The pleasures of the Wu Wei now belong to the adept who has entered the realm of heaven.

### Scripture of the Foundation of the Tao on Expelling and Taking In (Daojia Tuna Jing) (Seventh century CE)

This text also comments on the early side effects of fasting such as weakness, yellow color, dizziness, clumsiness, and weight loss. It, too, encourages the adept (with much risk) to push through these initial obstacles, claiming that this phase lasts for thirty days only. Thereafter strength, color, and vital energy return.[50] The table on page 201 summarizes these changes. Again the reader must realize that the feats accomplished by these immortals—if real—are incredible and that thirty days of fasting would often result in death today.

### Imbibing the Five Chis (Taishang Lingbao Wu Fu Xu) (Third century CE)[51]

This treatise presents various formulas that have some similarities to the Kan and Li practice, including formulas for absorbing the essence of the sun, moon, and Pole Star. Like the Universal Healing Tao Kan and Li practice, the fasting regime in this text is enabled by imbibing chi—which acts as a natural appetite suppressant—from Heaven and Earth. The book also mentions tips such as sucking on a jujube seed (Suan Zao Ren)[52] to ward off hunger. In traditional Chinese medicine, the jujube seed tonifies heart yin and therefore allays heart anxieties and calms the spirit.[53] The appetite suppression may therefore be in part due to the adept's being more tranquil and not disturbed by transitory hunger signals.

## SIDE EFFECTS OF FASTING

| FASTING DURATION | EFFECTS |
|---|---|
| 10 days | Fever, exhausted and yellow appearance |
| 20 days | Poor coordination, dizziness, weakness, aches and pains, constipation, dehydration, weight loss |
| 30 days | Emaciation, difficulty walking |
| 40 days | First signs of breakthrough: improved mood, mind settling |
| 50 days | Adept feels organs have good energy and luster, lower tan tien full of chi |
| 60 days | Muscle strength returns |
| 70 days | Continuing desire to avoid social contact and to meditate with astral flight |
| 80 days | Calm with tranquil emotions |
| 90 days | Facial appearance is smooth and glowing |
| 100 days | Three tan tiens full of chi |
| 3 years | Moles, burns, and scars disappear |
| 6 years | Supernatural powers of clairvoyance, healing, and the ability to dematerialize |
| 9 years | Ability to command supernatural beings: immortal status |

### Other Fasting Methods

Various other treatises of the Tao canon cite other methods of supporting fasting including ritual and talisman use. A ritual command can be verbally made to the appropriate deities, or a paper talisman can be ingested. The words "Do not allow me to thirst or hunger"[54] are repeated every day for sixty days facing the east.

# HERBS

Herbs were taken during Kan and Li retreats in ancient times for the following reasons:

1. To help heal preexisting underlying organ disease,
2. To help ward off hunger and act as an appetite suppressant,
3. To assist with the quest for immortality.

While herbs are a helpful adjunct to the retreat diet, there are dangers inherent in pursuing them. Liu I-Ming mentions that in his experience, adepts would become distracted in their pursuit of the perfect herb mixture. He says, "What they did not realize was that material medicines can only cure physical ailments and cannot cure immaterial ailments. Immaterial sickness can only be cured by gathering the primordial, true, unified energy."[55] This quest is similar to that in External Alchemy where all energies were mistakenly focused on preparing the Golden Elixir substance. Adepts should be focused on accessing higher levels of meditation—not on the herbs, nor the fasting, for that matter.

Despite the risks of becoming overly focused on herbs, they may nevertheless be useful to the current aspiring adept. Of course, if a student has medical problems, any prescribed herbs and Western medicines should be continued throughout the Tao Garden Dark Room retreat. The student may cautiously continue the Pi Gu diet with appropriate qualified medical support.

Unfortunately, the task of evaluating the plethora of herbs purported to have healing qualities or to assist in fasting is mind-boggling. In our capitalist world it is hard to determine the efficacy of such herbs as everyone wants to sell their product! Therefore we will provide the student with an overview of how to assess the usefulness of such herbs.

## Evaluation of Herbal Remedies from a Western Perspective

Western medicine attempts to justify therapies based on evidence. Evidence can be high or low quality. Sometimes evidence is lacking and the reason for justifying a treatment modality is based on expert opinion or anecdotal reports.

High-quality evidence involves large randomized trials. Ideally, these trials are double-blind, meaning the researchers and subjects are both unaware of which treatment is being used. Low-quality evidence involves smaller numbers, trials that are not randomized or blinded, and trials sponsored by agents that have pecuniary interest in the drug or herb.

There are standard ways of grading the evidence for any particular herb, as shown in the list below.

> **Level I:** Evidence obtained from at least one properly designed randomized controlled trial.
>
> **Level II-1:** Evidence obtained from well-designed controlled trials without randomization.
>
> **Level II-2:** Evidence obtained from well-designed cohort or case-control analytic studies, preferably from more than one center or research group.
>
> **Level II-3:** Evidence obtained from multiple time series with or without the intervention. Dramatic results in uncontrolled trials might also be regarded as this type of evidence.
>
> **Level III:** Opinions of respected authorities, based on clinical experience, descriptive studies, or reports of expert committees.[56]

### Problems of the Evidence-Based Approach

One of the major obstacles to the evidence-based approach is the fact that herbal companies and complementary institutions generally do not have the infrastructure or financial support to run huge trials. This is changing, however, and we do see mainstream literature appearing from time to time about remedies like echinacea for treating viral infections.

Further problems exist in that the goal of herbs during a Pi Gu diet is only for a select few people. Research occurs for common large-scale conditions such as weight loss, treatment of infections, and so on. For example, I (Andrew Jan) doubt if anyone would do a study on the efficacy of Ling Zhi fungus in obtaining a mystical experience for reclusive monks.

Therefore the justification of many herbs would be in the realm of expert opinion. For example, if a master says that a particular herb is efficacious, that would be classified as level III evidence only. This may have some credibility for you if that master has accomplished something that you personally want.* However, it is important to realize that any actual evidence is likely to be low-grade, anecdotal, and a matter of expert opinion only. If you ask ten different experts on one matter you will likely get ten different opinions. Nevertheless, in support of expert opinion, the reader is encouraged to explore the use of herbal supplements and fasting with the assistance of a qualified herbalist *and* to critically examine the evidence before undertaking the use of any particular herb or dietary recommendation. Each herbal and dietary regime should be examined not only for its potential benefits but also for its potential harm. These potentialities can be quantified as the Number Needed to Treat (number of patients required for one patient to receive the stipulated benefit) and the Number Needed to Harm (number required to have one adverse event).

---

*Tony Robbins, a popular New Age speaker, says, "If you want to be successful, find someone who has achieved the results you want and copy what they do and you will achieve the same results."[57]

Evidence-based medicine helps us evaluate various therapeutic modalities by demonstrating whether the Number Needed to Treat (for the benefits obtained) outweighs the Number Needed to Harm. It helps us answer the questions that patients present to practitioners, such as exploring a partial fasting regime, as they negotiate their health and illness. For example, doctor Michael Mosley has created a fasting regime consisting of two nonconsecutive days. On those fasting days you are allowed 500 calories. He provides sample fast-day menus in his book *The Fast Diet*.[58] There is some evidence that this diet regime is as effective as a continual caloric-restrictive diet.[59] The continual caloric-restrictive diet has already been shown to reduce breast cancer in women. Now there is evidence to suggest (though only from animal models) that intermittent fasting may do so also.[60] Research on heart disease (again in women) shows that intermittent fasting may be cardio-protective.[61] In a study of healthy older adult men, intermittent fasting was found to have a positive effect on the following metrics: body weight, body mass index, fat percentage, fat mass, blood pressure, total cholesterol, low-density lipoprotein cholesterol, and DNA damage.[62] Andreas Michalsen, in "Prolonged Fasting as a Method of Mood Enhancement in Chronic Pain Syndromes," a paper that reviews clinical evidence, says:

> Recent evidence from clinical trials shows that medically supervised modified fasting (200–500kcal nutritional intake/day) with periods from 7–21 days is efficacious in the treatment of rheumatic diseases and chronic pain syndromes. Here fasting is frequently accompanied by increased alertness and mood enhancement. The beneficial claims of fasting are supported by experimental research, which has found fasting to be associated with increased brain availability of serotonin, endogenous opioids, and endocannabinoids.[63]

Another review paper in the journal *Psychiatry Research* reports on a small but well-randomized trial as well as other controlled trials (level

I and II evidence) on the impact of fasting. Fasting in these trials lasted mostly up to ten days (but some protocols lasted up to three weeks) with caloric intakes less than 500 kcal, the use of gentle laxatives, and fluids of 2–3 liters per day. The authors conclude, "Clinicians have found that fasting was frequently accompanied by an increased level of vigilance and a mood improvement, a subjective feeling of well-being, and sometimes of euphoria. Therapeutic fasting, following an established protocol, is safe and well tolerated."[64]

Thus there is emerging Western medical evidence that prolonged medically supervised low-calorie fasting in durations similar to those prescribed in the dark room in Chiang Mai is beneficial in certain situations. It is the sort of research cited above that can help us investigate ancient methods and confirm benefits for students within a safe practice framework.

Medical investigations can often pick up evidence of harm before it becomes obvious in the clinical picture. Another review paper published in the *Western Journal of Medicine* states that "Medical complications seen in fasting include gout and urate nephrolithiasis, postural hypotension and cardiac arrhythmias." All these complications are serious and some are life-threatening. Thus potential harm exists with prolonged fasting.[65] This is why we advocate close qualified supervision with access to medical care and backed up by medical investigation. In Fond's review, when evaluating the shorter protocols (usually less than ten days duration) and administration of 500kcal as cited above, he found only the rare side effects of irritability, headache, fatigue, nausea, and stomach ache.[66] His contraindications for persons that shouldn't enter the fast included those with "eating disorders, a body-mass index below 20 or above 40, kidney or liver disease, gastric ulcer, severe comorbidities, including cancer, immunosuppressive premedication (except corticosteroids), alcoholism, psychosis, pregnancy, lactation, unexplained weight loss, and medication with diuretics (in order to avoid hyponatremia)."[67]

However, not all clinical circumstances or patients' questions are covered by evidenced-based trials. This would certainly apply to our example of finding the benefits of prolonged supervised fasting to improvement in meditation ability. To cover these gaps, health care practitioners must rely upon their own clinical experience, along with that of their colleagues. When making any decision on a particular management plan, the health care practitioner should fully inform the student of the evidence (or lack thereof) supporting the decision before the management plan (such as fasting for a meditation retreat) is embarked upon. A management plan should include references to evidence-based investigations that support the plan, while also citing their accuracy (sensitivity and specificity). A realistic treatment plan will also need to take into consideration the wishes, culture, and financial considerations of the patient.

The choice between alternative and mainstream investigations and therapies is often largely patient driven. However, a broad-minded health care practitioner, while having his or her own area of clinical expertise, would be willing to either refer or comanage a patient who expresses a wish for a blend of alternative and mainstream methods. It is both authors' wish that alternative and mainstream medicine would merge more fully, with the mainstream leading the amalgamation. The authors again warn readers about trying to use unproven ancient methods to improve their health and well-being. These ancient methods need to be superimposed upon current evidence and medical expertise to arrive at beneficial and safe outcomes.

Our aim in this chapter has been to highlight historical methods and theories while inspiring the reader to investigate them with caution and diligence. Devotees are always encouraged to read the classics to connect with Taoist masters of old. This, however, does not imply that we should blindly follow their methods. Dr. Andrew Jan is a Western-trained physician as well as a devoted Taoist practitioner. His aim is to bring the ancient practices forward such that spiritual illumination is achievable, yet to also keep the practices safe and avoid harm. The austere practices of the ancients are neither necessary nor appropriate in this modern world. This is easily seen with the ridiculous stone diets and the ingestion of poisonous chemicals recommended by External Alchemy in an effort to achieve immortality. Just because it's Taoist and ancient doesn't mean it's right! Likewise with severe fasting—it is not necessary! This may be because of the improved Kan and Li teaching and its modern-day understanding. Partial or complete fasting is a potentially dangerous procedure and not only should participants be medically screened, they should also be closely supervised and monitored by qualified personnel. Likewise the ingestion of herbs should be investigated and prescribed by a qualified herbalist who has completed a thorough history and examination and has performed relevant tests for the intended recipient. Readers that are inspired by techniques of the ancient heroes and immortals should attend the closely supervised dark room retreat at Tao Garden in Chiang Mai, Thailand. Readers should not commence partial fasting in isolation. In the Tao Garden, Master Mantak Chia—a modern-day Taoist master—presents a safe modern-day practice of partial fasting for a short finite period (maximum nineteen days), along with improved teachings of the Taoist meditations of yesteryear to assist students in obtaining the enlightenment of Kan and Li practice.

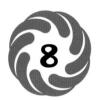

# Home Practice
## Embryo to Full Gestation

*But if one knows how to fill the belly and also empty
the mind, practices non-doing and incubates a spiritual
embryo, ever correct and undivided, using the natural
true fire to melt away the residual mundanity of acquired
conditioning, such a one is called the true human without
taint—how could regret not vanish? This is gathering in
the sense of incubating the spiritual embryo.*

LIU I-MING[1]

This chapter is for the advanced practitioner wishing to take her embryo
to full gestation and raise a spiritual body. Remember that the "embryo" is
a term to describe *your sense of the primordial within your tan tien and the
rest of your body*. It is a metaphor for aiding the understanding of the indescribable processes of this high level of meditation. The aim is to move
from an episodic sense of fullness in the tan tien to one that is permanent.
The rest of the body and mind will easily recall the wonderful primary
sensations of being in the womb. In other words, our aim is to congeal the
embryo state of being! Previously it was only to glimpse it! Now this state
of being stays with you forever.

The goal has shifted now from merely achieving health to that of
seeking enlightenment. It is about completing the gestation of the embryo

and raising a spiritual body. It takes a modicum of effort to conceive an embryo, but it is a larger task to complete gestation. The embryo must be protected against danger and rest in goodness.

Danger happens when one strays away from the simple path and does something silly. The simple path is a life excluding fame, fortune, and material indulgence.[2] Much like a mother who changes her ways once she has conceived, the adept guarding his or her embryo avoids silly behavior, including violating any of the Eight Pillars of health (see below).

In the Taoist literature there are two significant time periods for gestation: a hundred days and ten lunar months. The first period is similar to the point in a physical pregnancy when the woman is confident that the pregnancy has stabilized. This occurs after the first trimester at around the one-hundred-day mark. Women will often only announce their pregnancy after this date, as the chances of miscarriage are high before then. The ten-month time period corresponds to the forty- to forty-two-week gestation of a normal physical pregnancy.

At the end of the gestation period, the embryo is born and begins its independent journeying. Initial travels out of the body are short, but with practice the times can be prolonged. In these outward journeys, the Yuan Shen (Primordial Spirit) gathers information and knowledge from parts of the universe as part of its education.[3]

For most adepts, the simple life can be more easily achieved on retreat, which reduces the chances of significant distractions and stresses. On retreat or in the dark room, heightened states of meditation can be relatively easy to achieve. This is the so-called "honeymoon phase," and conception is relatively easy during this time. The work, however, is to continue the open state amid everyday pressures: to complete gestation and raise a spiritual body. Unfortunately, there are no easy shortcuts for this work. It is a matter of changing many aspects of your life. Much of the work of protecting the embryo can be understood in terms of guarding the Eight Pillars of health.

# GUARDING THE EIGHT PILLARS

The Eight Pillars must be managed and guarded in order to avoid miscarriage and ensure a live birth.

## Work

In *The Practice of Greater Kan and Li,* we quoted the great masters and their advice for our work choices. Lu Dong-Pin advised us against making rash decisions about our working life. He said, "When occupations come to us, we must accept them; when things come to us we must understand them from the ground up."[4] In *Understanding Reality,* Chang Po-Tuan tells us, "Before you have refined the restored elixir, do not go into the mountains; in the mountains, nothing within or without is real knowledge. The ultimate treasure is in everyone. Perhaps it is just that the ignorant do not fully recognize it."[5]

In other words, appreciate where your internal spirits have taken you thus far on your journey. So much of what we do in our specific trades or professions is almost irrelevant. It is the attitude that is underneath our work and how we interact with others that is most important. Somehow the issues that have previously created tension and fatigue need to be looked at in a new light. The adept must find the way from "the ground up," and be healed in the process. With a genuine heart, you can work to undo the knots of mistaken conditioning in the earthly realm. After a while, the base feelings release the spiritual body rather than curtailing it. It's as if the alchemical cauldron is finally in balance. At this point, some of the dross in the world is needed for you not only to transform yourself but to transform others.

Nevertheless, do not get lost in work with gay abandon. Be mindful of your lower tan tien and keep awareness of it most of the time. Do all tasks and procedures with only 75 percent intensity, so there is room for the mind to have partial awareness of the embryo. Do not over exert yourself, as this will deplete the embryo and threaten the pregnancy.

## Emotional Life

The emotional life is reduced overall, yet still maintains balance and spontaneity. This reduction and relative inner quietude will help congeal the embryo. Through our basic practices of the Six Healing Sounds, we discover the yin and yang aspects of our emotional body stemming from the five organs. We soon realize that negative emotions are not negative at all: they are just the yang aspects of our emotional being. The trouble is that temporal conditioning resulted in us suppressing our negative emotions.

Our initial healing steps were to release our suppressed yang emotions. However, following that we should come to realize that there is nothing wrong with feeling angry, frightened, sad, worried, or rushed. It's a question of balance and correctness. Our bodies are blessed with an emotional existence and these emotions are there to enliven and protect us. Ultimately they guide us home. Emotions are an important part of the healthy functioning of the lower and middle tan tiens.

Imbalance occurs when we suppress our emotions or they become attached to false knowledge—i.e., misplaced values including status, materialism, and indulgence in the external senses. These misplaced values lead our emotions to become attached to objects rather than the immortal realm. To this point Liu says the aim is to reduce the "influence of thought and emotion related to objects."[6] And further, Li Dao-Chun says, "Always extinguish the stirring mind, do not extinguish the shining mind. The unstirring mind is the shining mind."[7] The unstirring mind is the right environment for fostering the embryo in the lower tan tien.

The path to a reduction in the emotional body requires both strength and flexibility. The strength is to live by your own inner values, not those displayed by most people. It does not mean to be emotionally sterile, as there still will be moments of displaying the yang emotions. Yet in large part, there is a spontaneous drift toward virtue and quietude. This drift is without force and there is less intellectual reflection. With less intellectual pondering, the belly fills; this heralds success with the ongoing pregnancy. This drift is called "drumming on bamboo, calling the tortoise (symbol of longevity), eating jade mushrooms, plucking the lute, summoning the phoenix (symbol of immortality), and drinking from the alchemical crucible."[8]

Remember that the fetus has no obvious emotion; it is in a blissful world beyond the mundane.[9] The mundane world begets the emotions. Thus the adept must find a solution to these seemingly incompatible states. The solution may lie in the adept discovering how to act and behave emotionally from the One. If an emotion arises from this space, it is true. If it arises from a fragmented space mixed with attachment to the material world, then it is damaging.

## Sleep and Rest

In *The Practice of Greater Kan and Li* we introduced the concept of the triad of states of mind: the everyday awake mind, the dream mind, and the meditation mind. As one progresses toward raising a spiritual body, these three states of mind merge, so that the stillness of meditation becomes the center, while the formulas form the connection to the dream and awake worlds. Similarly, dreams form a connection between the meditation and awake worlds. Ultimately, formulas are practiced in the dreamtime: then the three worlds begin to blur.

There are now two times of the day that the adept explores the spirit world; meditation time and sleep time. During meditation the Nine Spirits are merged back into the Original Spirit (Yuan Shen). Spirits beyond the body are also encountered during meditation, with a focus on high-level pure spirits such as the Three Pure Ones. During sleep, the adept negotiates the spirit world again. Wei Po-Yang says, "Sleep is the embrace of spirit."[10]

To fully embrace the dream world, the adept needs to both remember dreams and learn how to dream lucidly. Remember, the spirit body was developed from your material body to enter the realm of spirits. Below, we have reproduced the Lucid Dreaming formula from *The Practice of Greater Kan and Li.*

#  Lucid Dreaming Formula

The principle behind this meditation is to gather the spirit or essence from each organ and then merge them in the lower tan tien.

1. Begin by lying on your back. Focus your mind on the lower tan tien.
2. Summon the spirits residing in the organs by chanting their names in the order of the creation cycle: *Houhou* or *Shen* (heart), *Beibei* or *Yi* (spleen), *Yanyan* or *Po* (lungs), *Fu Fu* or *Zhi* (kidneys), and *Jianjian* or *Hun* (liver).[11] You can also gather the other four spirits from above the crown, the head, behind the knees, and below the feet.
3. Repeat the chanting and gathering until a bright light and warmth appear in the lower tan tien. Opening this place will automatically open the Microcosmic Orbit.
4. Coordinate your breathing with this meditation to assist the process: inhaling stimulates the kidneys and liver, while exhaling moves the heart and lungs to the centerpoint—the stomach and spleen.
5. Now you can begin to lucid dream. Roll over, preferably with the right side down, with the left hand over the top aspect of the upper thigh of a bent leg. The right hand is placed under the head or at second best under the pillow (fig. 8.1).
6. Bring the merged five spirits from the lower tan tien (you can also include the other four spirits) up to the heart, and then to the Crystal Palace (also known as the Divine Palace or Hall of Light). The

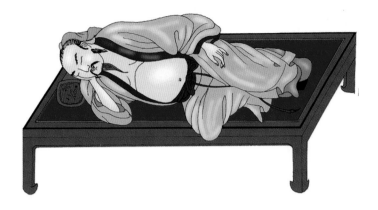

Fig. 8.1. The immortal Chen Tuan practicing
lucid dreaming in the classic dreaming posture

team of merged spirits—now the Yuan Shen or Original Spirit—
can exit via the crown.

7. Being conscious during the whole dream, or alternatively remembering the dream after waking, completes the process. You also have the
choice of practicing meditation during your dream state.

8. Process the content of the dream during the day, taking any actions in
the material world that are now necessary.

The adept should start to form a harmonious rhythm between the
three realms. Work should not interfere too much with this pattern, such
that "When tired I sleep, awake I act."[12] With the development of the
fetus, and with at least several hours of meditation per day, sleep requirements become less. The mind spends less time managing conflict between
the different spirits as they are all working together as a team. Chang Po-
Tuan says, "Sleep less and work more. Working by day, cautious by night,
effort never ceasing. Giving up sleep, forgetting to eat, the will must be
firm."[13]

Chang's tone is a bit too forceful here. Sleeping less happens spontaneously with practice. Likewise, eating will also reduce as the adept is

sustained more by chi and is less dependent on material foods. Ensuring success with the pregnancy involves being both gentle and spontaneous. Willpower alone—forcing less sleep and less food—will only result in failure.

## Sexuality

> *Do not be deluded by alcohol or sex. If you do not drink,*
> *your nature will not be deranged; if you are chaste, your*
> *life force will be stable.*
>
> CHANG PO-TUAN[14]

These are harsh words again from Chang Po-Tuan. For many, a life of chastity is unthinkable and would create a sense of violence if imposed. Sexuality is an important aspect of our being, which gradually becomes sublimated into our Kan and Li practice. To go from everyday sexuality to Dual Cultivation and finally Single Cultivation involves many steps and accomplishments. This takes years of devoted practice and certainly doesn't happen overnight. The harsher ascetic practices may be appropriate only for a chosen few. Those who choose it should let it happen of its own accord.

In the Universal Healing Tao system, the process of sublimating the sexual energy into the body is a long and complex one, which began with practices such as Ovarian and Testicular Breathing, the Power Lock, and the Orgasmic Upward Draw (fig. 8.2). In the Kan and Li practices, we also learned the techniques of self-intercourse (coupling), seeding, and pregnancy.

Early in our sexual lives, we search for that blissful mind, heart, and sexual feeling connection. Most of us need to learn the nature and rewards of sexual union in the material plane with a loving partner. Men can learn and practice the skills of semen retention. Being motivated by a loving heart is more powerful than the egotistical ideal of narcissistic self-mastery. Being soft, delicate, loving, and caring outweigh any notion

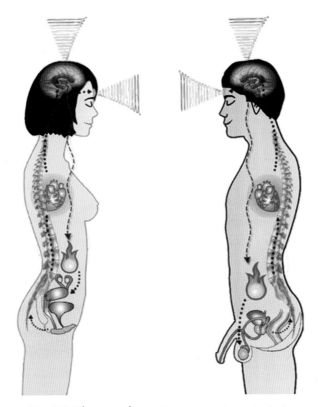

Fig. 8.2. The sexual practices are an important step
on the journey to mastering Kan and Li.

of self-indulgence. For women, it is important to put aside the primitive urge for procreation and drawing out of the male's semen to find a new rhythm that encourages mutual spiritual evolution. The female also finds the energetic drainage of menses tiring and moves herself to a different energetic level.

Both partners soon discover the arrows and stings of a long-term relationship and the darker aspects of the husband-wife law (Control Cycle) and return to the unconditional love of the Creation Cycle. With time these and many issues are solved and their lessons duly learned.

At an internal level, the consequence of sublimating sexual feelings is that sexual desire is gratified within the three tan tiens. This means that practitioners may have less need to explore the outside world to meet this desire. In Taoist practice, the mystical path is not restricted to celibates alone but exists for couples as well; however, the practice for adepts has the potential to create a naturally-found celibacy. The internal reality has complete sexual freedom within the constraints of the Inner Alchemical framework. All feelings and desires of the human person are deemed to have a purpose and are oriented toward the experience of Oneness.

In using sexual feelings to form mystical consciousness, the adept can learn to control sexual desire without meeting this desire externally (including ejaculation for men) or in a destructive manner. The adept discovers and connects to the "inner child," and his love is both matured and amplified. The mind becomes integrated and connected to something beyond the self. Direct experience is the central truth resulting in the force that enacts healing change in the individual and then cascades through the collective.

Direct mystical experience gives the adept a new-found authority. Perhaps this may have more influence on healing humanity than moral codes alone. Likewise, the UHT system uses sexual feelings because they are vital at every stage of the alchemical process and are necessary to realize the ultimate goal—the unitive state of the nameless One. If the individual can integrate their fragmented parts and let go of their self-identity, then that is enough.

In the UHT system, sexual energy is a vital ingredient, catalyst, and part of the major elements contributing to the alchemical framework. In the first stage of sexual awakening, the UHT system is adamant that sexuality needs to be transformed into a positive framework. Sexuality is not a self-disgusted process that is often displayed as rushed and violent. It certainly shouldn't be confined only within the realm of erotica and negative emotions. Rather, sexuality is meant to be soft, joyous, and inviting—like a flower. The opening of the lower tan tien and spiritual pregnancy embody this nature. In some Taoist sects, the pregnancy is called the "Yellow Sprouts." Taking the embryo to full gestation is the "Secret of the Golden Flower."[15]

In the next stage of development, the adept learns to merge the heart with sexual feelings. The heart is the charm that can tame the potentially ravaging power of the sexual urge. This merging with sexual feeling requires a purified heart. The UHT teaches that sexual feelings, if added to another emotion, will amplify that emotion whether it is positive or negative. Therefore, in order to purify the heart, practitioners need to vent feelings like rage and hatred. To purify the heart, all the fiery emotions need to be gathered and collected, which is done via the practice of Fusion of the Five Elements. Sexual feelings are released in this process, then added to the heart to awaken the middle tan tien. The product of a merged pure heart and sexual feeling creates a sensation of compassion, which results in a sense of softening and control of the sexual urge. It is a step closer to the Original Chi of the unity state. Sexual energy added to the heart enables the removal of tension in and around it and the release of its spirit, the Shen.

Finally, sexual feelings are merged with the mind and upper tan tien. The mind has to both broaden and retreat to an equal status with the other two tan tiens. This merging includes the energies and mind functions of the other two minds or tan tiens. It also includes parts of mind attributed to the organs, such as willpower (kidneys), courage and the earthly soul (lungs), kindness and the floating soul (liver), and thinking (spleen).

The UHT practice involves turning the senses inward toward the imagination. Sexual feeling is close to the tactile sense as it pertains to arousing the whole body. In Fusion and later the Sealing of the Five Senses, senses are merged into one with sexual feeling. For this mystical tradition, the pleasures of sexual feelings fuse the fragmented mind and assist in unifying this tripartite model of the mind. Again, sexual feeling acts as a catalyst for fusing the individual's multiple psychophysical energies.

By coupling contrary states of experience, this practice goes beyond the fused minds or tan tiens to mystical consciousness. Sexual feelings contribute to coupling, which is the central theme of all of the higher alchemical practices. In this process sexual desire creates an orgasmic feeling that is projected inwardly during meditation. Using an imagined cauldron, opposite states are cooked until they dissolve into the nameless One.

In assisting full gestation of the spiritual embryo there will be ongoing coupling. This coupling is intimately connected with sexual feeling and desire (Ching Chi). Sexual desire and feelings are at the very root of our being. This root is both wonderful and fundamental to our alchemical success. In the ideal, the sexual urge gathers and amplifies the forces of the five elements, the eight forces, and all the subtle variations of yin and yang to one purpose. This one purpose is to congeal the primordial force and stabilize the spiritual embryo till full gestation. This embryo will become a spiritual being of ultimate perfection. Full of compassion and healing ability, this being becomes the medicine of the world. How could sexuality be considered evil or wrong in this sense?

However, in order to align all of these energies, the sexual desire needs to be channelled in one direction. This does not mean that if you are practicing alone that personal fantasies and past love affairs cannot arise. Intermediate fantasies that are beyond your direct involvement can be utilized. These may include gods and goddesses making love above. You can even imagine making love with a deity to produce the spiritual embryo! However, eventually these do dissipate and become untainted and pure. Unadulterated sexual desire fills the cauldron with yin and amplifies the fire beneath. As the dual forces merge, the end result becomes tangible and the spiritual infant arises with all its love and wisdom. The connection between your sexual drive and your spiritual body in all its beauty arises. Therefore you release deeper and deeper libidinous urges. It is only at the base of this seemingly endless abyss that the process will be complete.

For the adept who chooses single cultivation, the sexual urge is satisfied within. Love from the heart and the positive engagement of spirit is satisfying. Liu I-Ming says to this point: "When vitality [Kan/Ching Chi] is governed by the spirit, water is treated with fire and thoughts of lust disappear. . . . When lust disappears, the vitality is whole so the belly is full."[16] The material urge for encounters of the flesh naturally becomes reduced. There is no need for enforced discipline. This evolution and progress occurs without effort.

For those partaking in dual cultivation their sexuality takes on new meaning. Together, they strive for the same medicine. They love each other as much as they love their spiritual work. Healing flows from this couple as it would from any accomplished immortal.

## Other Pillars: Exercise, Water, and Healthy Spirituality

The Eight Pillars have been extensively discussed in our other works: *The Practice of Greater Kan and Li, Tai Chi Fa Jin,* and *Tai Chi Wu Style,* as well as in chapter 2 of this text. So we won't belabor the pillars of health here. While Kan and Li practice is an exercise and form of Chi Kung in itself, ideally it should be accompanied by Tao Yin, Chi Kung, and Tai Chi practice. Good water collected in nonpolluted surroundings is a must. Given that food becomes less important with high level practice, the quality of water and air both become more noticeable and important. Healthy spirituality is completely covered by Kan and Li practice.

## RETREAT PRACTICE

Ultimately, the serious adept needs time in retreat. Progress can only go so far while partaking in life within a community. To begin with, attend a one- or two-week retreat or workshop that allows sitting in meditation for at least six hours per day. In the cities, many Buddhist communities offer Vipassana retreats that include ten days of silent meditation. You may find it difficult, however, to practice Taoist meditation with the teacher directing you to be only mindful of your breath (Anapanasati). Some retreats offer complete isolation within a cell or room, which is even more ideal. Christian organizations also offer facilities for personal retreats. Taoist centers are gradually on the increase, so please explore your local region for various options. The Universal Healing Tao centers offer the opportunity not only for your own space but also for guidance on Kan and Li meditations.

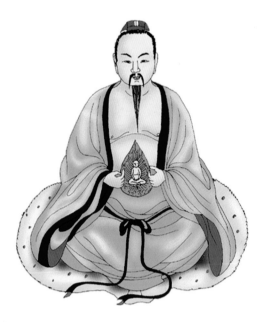

Fig. 8.3. After a hundred days of practice, the embryo should be formed and secure.

A couple of weeks may be enough to conceive, but it will not be enough to hold a pregnancy. Lu Dong-Pin urges adepts to embark on a hundred-day retreat. It is in a hundred days that the adept begins to understand the hourly chi cycle of a day and the variation of forces within a week. Lu Dong-Pin says that only a hundred-day retreat allows the adept enough time to truly practice self-intercourse and create the internal light, then circulate it according to the Wheel of the Law. At this stage, this light will be refined enough to be called "spirit fire."[17] Lu says, "When a person has found the method of making thoughts and energy harmonize with one another, he can complete the elixir within the hundred days (fig. 8.3)."[18] By the elixir he means formation of the embryo. By then, the experience will become solid and eventual birth of the spiritual infant very likely. However, Lu makes the proviso that if the adept is still recovering from illness then success is not guaranteed.

The next level is to embark on a retreat for ten lunar months. At this stage, the effects of the seasons upon the eight kuas are recognized. Life returns to utter simplicity allowing total devotion to immersion in the energetic worlds. Furthermore, a prolonged retreat of ten lunar months is intimately linked with the gestation period of an actual embryo in the material world.

It is possible, of course, that after some months of isolated practice an adept could theoretically continue training and the pregnancy while mingling in community life. However, a very strong will would be required. The working life would need to be simple. Many boundaries around social interactions would be required. Food, alcohol, coffee, and entertainment all provide ready-made distractions for such serious work. Teaching the Tao as much as possible may prove to be the antidote to such calamities.

As mentioned elsewhere, the embryo is signified by a permanent sense of primordial vibration and light in the tan tien. This energy not only fills the tan tien but is felt throughout the body and perceived by all the senses. This is opposed to a transient experience that can happen in a workshop or during daily meditation. In other words, the body has remained open enough for the permanent fusion of Kan and Li or Heaven and Earth's

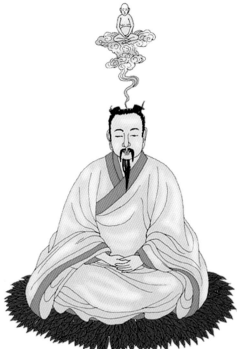

Fig. 8.4. After ten months in retreat the fetus should be mature and ready to form a spiritual body.

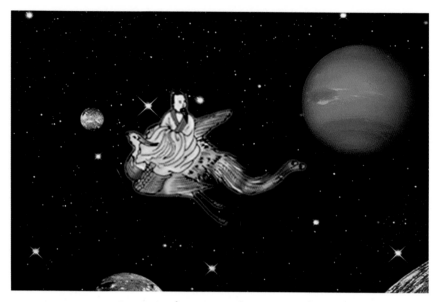

Fig. 8.5. After ten months in retreat the
adept can practice astral flight for prolonged periods.

energies in the Elixir Field. If these dualities can remain fused for a full
gestation period of ten lunar months, then we can say that the spiritual
body is fully formed and ready for astral flight (fig. 8.4). This created
energy ball is able to leave the body via the Central Thrusting Channel
and partake in astral flight (fig. 8.5).

In astral flight, the spiritual body gathers even more refined primordial essence, gaining an experience of nothingness, which corresponds to
deep outer space. As one reaches the vast emptiness, stillness pervades!
Breathing ceases and fetal respiration is almost permanent. The adept
appears to be in a state of hibernation. All duality is basically resolved
with time becoming one in the moment. The vastness of the universe is
experienced as one sensation. The observer's sense of self is totally lost
and there is no difference between the Tao and the adept. They are one!

For those ready to embark on years of isolation, *The Scripture of the
Foundation of the Tao on Expelling and Taking In* gives us an idea of what
to expect!

## BENEFITS OF PROLONGED RETREAT AND PRACTICE

| 100 days | Tan tien full of chi |
|---|---|
| 3 years | Moles, burns, and scars disappear |
| 6 years | Supernatural powers of clairvoyance, healing, and the ability to dematerialize |
| 9 years | Ability to command supernatural beings; immortal status[19] |

The challenge is to orchestrate your life in such a way that these long retreats become a regular reality. There are some senior instructors within our system who have set up such spaces for themselves. One owns his own mountain, while many have set up rural housing and retreats. If you can set this up you are to be congratulated. Kan and Li practice is a serious commitment for a select few. While daily practice is possible with Kan and Li, formation of the embryo and solid spiritual body formation require extreme devotion.

Life for the serious devotee becomes a mixture of isolation in nature and mixing with city life. Ultimately, the aim is "to live mingling in the world yet in harmony with the light."[20] Live in the world yet transcend the world. You have your retreats, yet join the community. You make decisions that subtly influence the evolution of mankind. Each one person affects only a few—but ultimately the vision of the One transcends fragmentation and exploitation. The single most powerful guidance is connection to this unitive state of mind.

For the individual who successfully mixes isolation and city life, there is a spontaneous return to the uncarved block. Ideally ideas arise from this space. Thoughts arise. There is no logic, no intellectual rigor—just what is natural. "When no idea arises, the right idea comes. That is the true idea," says Lu Dong-Pin.[21]

Allow your life to move away from status and expectation and instead move to an expanse centered in and governed by what arises from this primordial space. Remember that the primordial represents fusion of all parts—all have contributed their part. Nothing is forgotten and all is welcome. This is the space that should govern not only your life but also the lives of others.

"Becoming immortal" means giving up your mortal desire to satisfy the external five senses. To no longer relish the taste of fine foods. To enjoy feeling hungry and the taste of bitter and sour. Fine music goes out the door! The inner sounds of the tiger's *Ooommm* and the *Eeeeee* of the dragon's roar are loud enough. Even better is the sweet sound of silence. Silence exerts its rejuvenating echoes all the way to the soul. Visuals—movies—are okay but not as penetrating and healing as the inner light. Even better than the inner light is the comforting darkness of the Wu Wei. With time the adept appreciates that the primordial or the elixir is the one true goal. The elixir is so delicate, so pure, so healing—it is beyond anything else worthwhile describing. The paradox with all this is that once you have drunk this inner elixir then the outside world is so much more beautiful. Once you return to the source and become natural, fame may come but it occurs with no effort and through no act of wanting!

There is always a delicate balance of responsibilities and contribution to society. We recognize that we are part of the whole. Our individual identity is of less concern compared to the evolution of the planet. Individual responsibilities carry with them mental preoccupation. This mental preoccupation attempts to create solutions to problems that are often unsolvable. This distracts the mind and disturbs the appreciation of peace and tranquillity. Ge Hong was a great advocate of limiting responsibilities within society. Life is easiest as a simpleton, which is often one way of translating *Bao Pu Tzu*. Yet total appreciation of the peace and tranquillity at the center of all disturbances can obviate any desire to help others. Give too much and suffer the consequence. Staying isolated and denying being a part of the continuum is not being truly connected. The balance between the two is a matter of individual choice.

# Appendix

# *Major Classic Texts Pertaining to Kan and Li*

| DATE & PERIOD | TITLE | CHINESE TITLE | AUTHOR | ALCHEMICAL FOCUS | MODERN TRANSLATION |
|---|---|---|---|---|---|
| Second Century CE | *Instructions on the Scripture of the Divine Elixirs of the Nine Tripods by the Yellow Emperor* | Huangdi Jiuding Shendan Jingjue | Anonymous | External Alchemical text, but provides a framework for Inner Alchemical processes and nomenclature | Pregadio, Fabrizio. *Great Clarity: Daoism and Alchemy in Early Medieval China.* California: Stanford University Press, 2006. |
| Fourth Century CE | *The Master Who Embraces Simplicity* | Bao Pu Tzu | Ge Hong | Probably the most outstanding collection on Neidan and Weidan | Ware, James. *Alchemy, Medicine and Religion in the China of A.D. 320: The Nei P'ien of Ko Hung (Bao Pu Tzu)* NY: Dover Publications, 1981. |

## MAJOR TEXTS PERTAINING TO KAN AND LI (con't.)

| DATE & PERIOD | TITLE | CHINESE TITLE | AUTHOR | ALCHEMICAL FOCUS | MODERN TRANSLATION |
|---|---|---|---|---|---|
| 142 CE | *Triplex Unity* | Zhouyi Can Tong Qi | Wei Po-Yang | Poetical text highlighting the trigrams as a basis for alchemical formation of the Golden Elixir, includes the terms Gold Elixir, lead, mercury, dragon and tiger, medicines, fetus, cauldron | Bertschinger, Richard. *The Secret of Everlasting Life: The First Translation of the Ancient Chinese Text of Immmortality.* Rockport, MA: Element, 1994. |
| Probably Tang era | *Scripture of the Dragon and Tiger* | Longhu Jing | Unknown | The dragon and tiger become symbols of the interplay between Kan and Li or yin and yang in the return to the One and the Golden Elixir | Wong, Eva. *Harmonizing Yin and Yang: The Dragon-Tiger Classic.* Boston: Shambhala, 1997. |
| Tang era | *The Secrets of the Golden Flower* | Tai Yi Chin Hua Tsung Zhi | Lu Dong-Pin or students | Landmark text that blends some Buddhist with Taoist thought on Inner Alchemy; meditations represent a blend of the Microcosmic Orbit, Fusion, and Kan and Li practices | Wilhelm, Richard. Commentary by Carl Jung. *The Secrets of the Golden Flower: A Chinese Book of Life.* London: Routledge & Kegan Paul, 1975. |

| DATE & PERIOD | TITLE | CHINESE TITLE | AUTHOR | ALCHEMICAL FOCUS | MODERN TRANSLATION |
|---|---|---|---|---|---|
| Ninth Century | *The Teachings of the Tao as Transmitted by Chung and Lu* | Chung Lu Chuan Tao Chi | Lu Dong-Pin (or students) | Theories on Internal Alchemy and three paths to health, longevity, and immortality; text influenced both Quanzhen (Northern Complete Reality school) and Nanzong (Southern) | Wong, Eva. *The Teachings of Immortals Chung and Lu: The Tao of Health and Longevity, and Immortality.* Boston: Shambhala, 2000. |
| 1075 CE | *Awakening to Reality* | Wu Zhen Pian | Chang Po-Tuan | Chang uses poetical language to assist the adept with Internal Alchemy. However, it is the commentary by Liu I-Ming that consolidates the ideas. Together they work well to improve the reader's understanding. | Cleary, Thomas. *Understanding Reality: A Taoist Alchemical Classic.* Honolulu: University of Hawaii Press, 1987. |
| Eleventh Century | *Understanding Reality & Four Hundred Character Treatise on the Gold Elixir (Inner Teachings of Taoism)* | Jin Dan Si Bai Zi | Chang Po-Tuan | Again commentary provided by Liu I-Ming | Cleary, Thomas. *The Inner Teachings of Taoism.* Boston: Shambhala, 2001. |
| Thirteenth Century | *The Book of Balance and Harmony* | Zhong He Ji | Li Dao-Chun | Collection of Internal Alchemy teachings from the Complete Reality school | Cleary, Thomas. *The Book of Balance and Harmony.* Boston: Shambhala, 1989. |

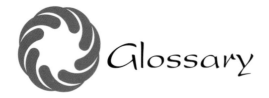# Glossary

**Bao Pu Tzu (Bao Pu Zi, Pao Pu Tzu):** *The Master Who Embraces Simplicity* written by Ge Hong (283–343 CE). Joseph Needham described Ge Hong as the greatest alchemist in Chinese history. The Inner Chapters are concerned with alchemy, while the Outer Chapters are on Confucian subjects.

**breathing, fetal:** A breathing pattern that simulates the breathing of the fetus in the womb. This includes two phenomena: the first is that there is no external obvious movement of the chest or the sound of the breath with respiration. From an experiential and medical perspective, subtle air exchange may occur despite the absence of external visible signs. The second is that the practitioner begins to swallow saliva, like a fetus swallowing amniotic fluid. "He who can breathe like a fetus will respire as if still in the womb, without using nose or mouth; thus the Tao will be achieved."[1]

**breathing, immortal:** A term used by Charles Luk associating Turning of the Wheel not only with cessation of external signs of respiration but also with absence of a physical pulse. Internally the adept is likely to be in a deep trance state, completely merging with the Wu Wei.

**cauldron (furnace):** The cauldron is the tool required to couple fire and water. The lower tan tien is the biggest and made of clay. The solar plexus cauldron is made of iron and can withstand very hot fire. The heart tan tien is made of jade and requires purified heat and steam to heat the purified water. The coupling in the head is inside the Crystal Palace and is even more delicate. The heavenly furnace is made of gold.

**coupling (self-intercourse):** The forces of Kan and Li, yin and yang, and dragon and tiger become merged through a process akin to sexual intercourse. The forces engage, thrust, and penetrate. The intercourse creates intense and at times pleasurable pain with accompanying blissful sensations and emotions. The two forces merge to lose their old identity and become something new. Coupling can lead to orgasm and even internal ejaculation resulting in conception of an immortal fetus.

**court (chamber):** Yellow Court (Huang Ting) is the center of the human being, gate of all wonders or gate of nondual doctrine. In the *Scripture of the Yellow Court,* it appears to correspond to the spleen.[2] It is my impression [Andrew Jan] that the several texts refer to the solar plexus cauldron as the Yellow Court. Either way, given the variation in meaning, the Yellow Court is the cauldron where yin and yang or Kan and Li forces meet to produce a merged refined elixir. Yellow is usually used to denote gold, which implies the primordial essence.

**cinnabar:** A term used in External Alchemy. Red cinnabar is a stone that contains mercuric oxide. In Internal Alchemy this stone symbolizes the heart. Mercury symbolizes the yang dragon arising in the house of Li.

**dragon:** Metaphor for the vapor or chi that arises from the heart but originally from the liver, and manifests itself in the house of Li. It is outwardly yang energy that arises out of the heart fire. The *Eeeee* sound of the dragon is like a high frequency sound that originates from the heavens. Once the dragon is coupled with the tiger, its yin nature is revealed as the "grease of dragons" that correlates to mercury in External Alchemy.

**dynasties, duration of:**

| Dynasty | Years |
|---|---|
| Zhou | 1046–256 BCE |
| Spring and Autumn Period | 722–476 BCE |
| Warring States | 476–221 BCE |
| Qin | 221–206 BCE |
| Han | 206 BCE–220 CE |
| Three Kingdoms | 220–265 CE |
| Jin | 265–420 CE |
| Southern and Northern | 420–589 CE |
| Sui | 581–618 CE |
| Tang | 618–907 CE |
| Five and Ten Kingdoms | 907–960 CE |
| Song | 960–1279 CE |
| Liao | 916–1125 CE |
| Yuan | 1271–1368 CE |
| Ming | 1368–1644 CE |
| Qing | 1644–1911 CE |

**elixir:** The term connotes healing and therefore has overlap with terms such as *medicine* or *pill*. In External Alchemy it represents the merging of base elements into an alchemical elixir that can be ingested to cause healing, longevity, or immortality. In Internal Alchemy, elixir represents an essence that results from purification or merging of variant energies such as the five elements, the eight forces, three fields (San Bao, Ching Chi, and Shen), dualities such as Kan and Li, or the spiritual with the mundane. There are various types of elixir.

**Elixir, Golden (Chin Tan):** Is the product of the fusion of the basic duality of yin and yang to form the Primordial Chi, essence, or observation (Yuan Cheu). This can be experienced in a tan tien or via the third eye. Alternatively it is the merging of the spirit (Shen) with the generative force (Ching Chi). The latter implies the mixture of external light with internal sexual feeling.

**Elixir, Jade:** Purified essence from the upper cauldron returning to the lower tan tien.

**essence:** A confusing term that in practical experiential terms implies an inner sensation that gives the impression of solidity and purity (movement to the primordial). Chi is often felt as gaseous while essence is a more solid liquid sensation. When chi is purified or merged with other variant energies there is a reversal of the creation sequence and a march toward unity.[3] With practice, chi can be refined, merged, and condensed to produce essence. Elixir and essence have overlap in meaning, except elixir connotes healing. The Chinese term *tan* can mean either essence or elixir. However, scholars such as Pregadio prefer the former.[4]

**fangshi:** Alchemical practitioner.

**fetus (embryo):** A state whereby chi in the lower tan tien is continually present. In the nonpregnant state the lower tan tien can be formed but disappears when in everyday tasks. The sensation is that the lower tan tien is continually vibrating or spinning. One can use sexual metaphors to describe progress in these inner esoteric alchemical arts. The pregnant state results from self-intercourse, with merging of all aspects of self and insemination of spirit from the spleen, liver, or the heavens. When mature, the fetus leaves the body via the Central Thrusting Channel through the crown. After leaving the crown it becomes the spiritual body, which can fly to the heavens.

**furnace:** *See* cauldron

**gold (yellow):** In External Alchemy gold represents the goal of the chemical practice, in which base metals such as lead, mercury, tin, or iron are transmuted into the prize metal of gold. In Internal Alchemy, gold also represents the prized experiential state. Gold is equated with pleasant, smooth, and blissful sensations. While gold connotes a yellow color with this metaphor, in reality the adept may not experience this color. In many classical texts the term *yellow* (*huang*) is used. Yellow also signifies a higher purified and merged state. Terms such as the Golden Elixir, Golden Pill, Yellow Sprouts (flowers), Yellow Court, and Yellow Old Man[5] all imply a prized state.

**ghost (*kuei*):** A term used to describe spirit entities that are not benevolent and are associated with the realms of the earth or hell. It is alleged that a ghost can result from poor or absent spiritual practice. Ghosts have no name and are yin. Like concepts in Buddhism, kuei can choose to enter the human realm again. The concepts of kuei are not a feature of modern practice and are more indicative of older sects such as Shanqing Taoism.

**Huai Nan Tzu (*The Sages of the Huai Nan*):** A Taoist/Confucian text from the Han period ~ 200 BCE written by Prince Liu An of Huai Nan, which includes foundation theories of yin and yang and the five elements.

**Huang Ting:** *See* Yellow Court

**Hun Ho:** Merging into Oneness (Inner Alchemy)—a Shanqing (Mao Shan) practice that is closely related to the Universal Healing Tao practice of Fusion.

**I Ching:** The Book of Changes that Taoist alchemists used to define the path and the nature of interaction between yin and yang. The ideal Taoist path was to cultivate the way of Heaven (immortality) by embracing (repelling) Earth.[6]

**Kan (trigram of water):** The trigram of yin-yang-yin. It includes the symbol of the jade rabbit in the moon (yang). It houses the yin tiger that is heard as the eternal sound: *Ooommm.*

**lead:** A term used in both Internal and External Alchemy. In External Alchemy lead was supposedly transformed into silver. This may have just been purified untarnished molten lead. In Internal Alchemy, black lead corresponds to the kidney and silver corresponds to the yin tiger manifesting itself in the house of Kan. True Lead corresponds to purified lead and represents the first stage in extracting Kan energy. In the Quanzhen tradition it represents true vitality, which is felt as purified Ching or generative Chi.

**Li (trigram of fire):** The trigram of yang-yin-yang. In Internal Alchemy it includes the symbol of the Dark Raven (black spot of the sun). Li houses the dragon with its high-pitched *Eeeeee* sound that rebounds through the ages of man. In External Alchemy Li corresponds to the compound cinnabar.

**medicine (pill):** The elixir that results from the intercourse (copulation) of Kan and Li (dragon and tiger). This elixir becomes the Great Medicine because it involves a merging of higher magnitude. Higher magnitude implies that Li can be represented by distant light from far away with the inner purified water essence. In historical senses this might be the result of approximately nine years' work. The Lesser Medicine (Pill) is of a lower quality compared to the Great Medicine because the depth of the interaction of Kan and Li is of a lower degree and involves approximately three years of Inner Alchemical work.

**mercury (quicksilver):** Used as a heavy metal in External Alchemy. It can be used in its oxide form initially as red cinnabar that supposedly would form the reduced metallic form. In Internal Alchemy, the purification of Li would release mercury symbolized as the "grease of dragons."

**Mysterious Pass:** This is the point between which yin and yang arise or merge, i.e., the point between Kan and Li. This has no fixed anatomical point and can occur in the tan tien or via a vision in the third eye, often described as the "inner eye." It is where all things converge and arise. It is related to the Primordial Chi and is one of its many guises.

**Ni Wan:** The Muddy Palace between the third eye and Jade Pillow. It is experienced as soft, pleasant, and mushy when meditating. Some cite the top of the crown as Ni Wan.

**Nei Dan:** The Practice of Inner Alchemy, this is opposed to Wei Dan (External Alchemy). *Dan* (Tan) can also be translated as "essence" or "elixir."

**Quanzhen school:** Complete Reality school.

**Sacred Ground:** The roof of the palate. The saliva above the tongue is called the Heavenly Pool and the connection is called another Mysterious Gate.

**spirit:** Usually implies consciousness outside of the body. There are various levels of spirit that can animate a body or exist independently. For the sincere adept the purpose is to practice so as to become a high-level spirit. Spirit and immortality are closely related states of being. Becoming immortal initially involves developing one's original spirit (Yuan Shen). The Yuan Shen's goal is to leave the body and merge with the Wu Wei. Yuan Shen is formed by the fusion of the virtues of the spirits of the five organs—Po, Hun, Zhi, Yi, and Shen. Yuan Shen manifests itself as spontaneous, ever changing, and arising from no self. There is no attachment to habit, the senses, or earthly desires. There is freedom from the anxieties and fears of everyday mortals. Low or incomplete spirits include persons who have not commenced or only partially entertained spiritual practice. The everyday undeveloped shen resides in the heart, while the Yuan Shen is located in its original "Cavity of the Spirit" (Yuan Shen Shih) located in the Crystal Palace.

**Sung:** To relax (Fa Sung).

**silver:** A higher grade metal. In External Alchemy it is derived from black lead. In Internal Alchemy silver arises from the purification of Kan.

**sulphur:** A base ingredient used in External Alchemy. It has no consistent correspondent in Internal Alchemy.

**Tao Chia Taoism:** Philosophical Taoism.

**Taiqing sect:** Great Clarity movement that prioritized External Alchemy.

**tiger:** Metaphor for the vapor or chi that arises from the kidneys that was originally from lungs and manifests itself in the house of Kan. It is yin energy externally but yang internally. The roar of the tiger is an *Ooommm* sound that is experienced from the earth.

**Wheel of the Law (Fa Lun)/Waterwheel:** This Wheel of the Law is closely linked to the Waterwheel. The Waterwheel in turn marks the Microcosmic Orbit. Both provide metaphors to aid understanding of this fundamental principle. The best aid to interpretation is a chapter devoted to its description in *The Teachings of Immortals Chung and Lu,* whereby Lu states the Law as the fundamental principle of the universe with the Law being "patterned after the structure of the sky and earth."[7] Basically everything spins like a wheel. In order to arrive at the elixir or the Tao one must spin the wheel. The wheel ensures that all energies are mixed and merged to enable reversal of the cosmological sequence and arrive at the goal (Wu Wei). There are two obligations to this wheel: one is that it starts with water and the second is that the wheel is driven by coupling in the respective tan tiens. Grades of the Waterwheel include the Smaller, the Greater, and the Purple

Waterwheel. The Smaller Waterwheel involves Fusion of the Five Elements while the Greater Waterwheel involves copulation of Kan and Li including the dragon and tiger to produce the Great Medicine. The Purple Waterwheel is the highest level, with mixing of the Golden Elixir until the body has disappeared and mystical vision of the Tao has occurred.[8]

**Wei Dan:** External Alchemy.

**Wu Wei:** State of nothingness or oneness associated with the merging of yin and yang. Can be used to describe a state of mind in parallel with the Taoist creation story.

**Yellow Court (Huang Ting):** The Yellow court is the center of the human being, gate of all wonders or gate of non-dual doctrine. In the *Scripture of the Yellow Court,* it appears to correspond to the spleen.[9] I is our impression that the several texts refer to the solar plexus cauldron as the Yellow Court. Either way, given the variation in the meaning, the Yellow Court is the cauldron where yin and yang or Kan and Li forces meet to produce a merged refined elixir. Yellow is usually used to denote gold, which implies the primordial essence.

**Yellow Old Man:** The observer of the cauldron.

**Yellow Sprouts:** Again this has some overlap with the Golden Elixir and Primordial Force but represents the basic life force which is sensed once temporal conditioning (false knowledge) is removed.

**Yellow Woman:** That state of meditation which facilitates easy union between Kan and Li. The term may have been used by male practitioners because of its soft, sensual, and soothing nature, which has some overlap with the Golden Elixir.

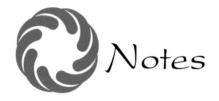

# Notes

## Chapter 1.
## Taoist History Related to the Greatest Kan and Li Meditation

1. Chang Po-Tuan and Liu I-Ming in Cleary, trans., *The Inner Teachings of Taoism,* 62.
2. Lao-tzu in Kwok, trans., *Tao de Ching,* 45.
3. Lao-tzu in Feng and English, trans., *Tao Te Ching,* verse 10.
4. Pregadio, *Great Clarity: Daoism and Alchemy,* 213.
5. Wong, *Taoism: A Complete Introduction,* 62.
6. Ibid., 63.
7. Ettington, *Immortality: A History and How To Guide,* 40
8. Ruan Fang-Fu, *Sex in China,* 56.
9. Ge Hong in Campany, trans., *To Live as Long as Heaven and Earth,* 178.
10. Pregadio, ed., *The Encyclopedia of Taoism,* vol. 1, 813–18.
11. Esposito, "Longmen Taoism in Qing China," 198.
12. Pregadio, ed., *The Encyclopedia of Taoism,* vol. 1, 815.
13. Esposito, "Longmen Taoism in Qing China," 191.
14. Ibid.
15. Ibid., 198.
16. Ibid., 192.
17. Ibid., 212.
18. Ibid.
19. Komjathy and Kang Siqi, *Daoist Texts in Translation,* www.daoistcenter.org/texts.pdf (accessed July 2011).
20. Winn, "Daoist Internal Alchemy in the West," 190.
21. Miller, *Chinese Religions in Contemporary Societies,* 268.
22. Winn, "Daoist Internal Alchemy in the West," 194.
23. Winn, *Journal of Daoist Studies,* vol. 2, 2009, http://threepinespress.com/?p=6.

24. Kohn, "Guarding the One," 126.
25. Ibid., 141.
26. Ibid., 130.
27. Ibid., 139.
28. Ibid., 132.
29. Ibid., 147. Bracketed text added by the authors.
30. Robinet, *Taoist Meditation*, 107.
31. Ibid., 105.
32. Ibid., 113.
33. Girardot, *Myth and Meaning in Early Taoism*, 358.
34. Lu Dong-Pin in Wong, trans., *The Teachings of Immortals Chung and Lu,* 104.
35. Chen Kai-Guo and Zheng Shun-Chao in Cleary, trans., *Opening the Dragon Gate,* 53, 82.
36. Miller, *Chinese Religions in Contemporary Societies,* 268.
37. Wong in Wong, trans., *The Teachings of Immortals Chung and Lu,* 11.
38. Chen Kai-Guo and Zheng Shun-Chao in Cleary, trans., *Opening the Dragon Gate,* 82.
39. Ibid., 53.

# Chapter 2.
## Why Practice the Greatest Kan and Li Meditation?

1. Chang Po-Tuan and Liu I-Ming in Cleary, trans., *The Taoist Classics,* vol. 2, 150.
2. Emoto, *The True Power of Water.*
3. Mantak Chia, see: www.universal-tao.com/article/supplementary.html.
4. Ibid.
5. Liu I-Ming in Cleary, trans., *The Inner Teachings of Taoism,* 13.
6. Ibid., 12.
7. Blake, *The Complete Poetry and Prose of William Blake,* 1.
8. Wittgenstein, *Tractatus Logico-Philosophicus* 6.431, available online: www.kfs .org/~jonathan/witt/t6431en.html.
9. Ge Hong in Campany, trans., *To Live as Long as Heaven and Earth,* 178.
10. Olsen, *The Jade Emperor's Mind Seal Classic,* 13.
11. Lu Dong-Pin and Chung Li-Chuan in Wong, trans., *The Teachings of Immortals Chung and Lu,* 26–30.
12. Ibid., 110.
13. Ibid., 27.
14. Ibid., 32.
15. Wong, trans., *The Teachings of Immortals Chung and Lu,* 15.

16. Lu Dong-Pin and Chung Li-Chuan in Wong, trans., *The Teachings of Immortals Chung and Lu,* 110.

17. Wei Po-Yang in Wu and Davis, trans., "An Ancient Chinese Treatise on Alchemy," 261.

18. Wong, trans., *The Teachings of Immortals Chung and Lu,* 15

19. Lu Dong-Pin in Wilhelm, trans., *The Secrets of the Golden Flower,* 58.

20. Wong, trans., *The Teachings of Immortals Chung and Lu,* 102.

21. Ge Hong in Campany, trans., *To Live as Long as Heaven and Earth,* 59.

22. Ibid., 109, 275, 308, and 344.

# Chapter 3.
# Principles of the Greatest Kan and Li Meditation

1. Li Dao-Chun in Cleary, trans., *The Taoist Classics,* vol. 2, 451.

2. Chang Po-Tuan and Liu I-Ming, in Cleary, trans., *The Inner Teachings of Taoism,* 8.

3. Ibid., 100.

4. Ibid., 60.

5. Ibid., 101.

6. Wong, *The Shambhala Guide to Taoism,* 183.

7. Chang Po-Tuan and Liu I-Ming in Cleary, trans., *The Inner Teachings of Taoism,* 100.

8. Chang Po-Tuan and Liu I-Ming in Cleary, trans., *Taoist Classics,* vol. 2, 139.

9. Chang Po-Tuan and Liu I-Ming in Cleary, trans., *The Inner Teachings of Taoism,* 57.

10. Ibid., 11.

11. Cleary, comp and trans., *Taoist Meditation,* 121.

12. Chang Po-Tuan and Liu I-Ming in Cleary, trans., *Taoist Classics,* vol. 2, 54.

13. Chang Po-Tuan and Liu I-Ming in Cleary, trans., *The Inner Teachings of Taoism,* 102.

14. Preservers of Truth sect from the Complete Reality school in Cleary, trans., *Taoist Classics,* vol. 2, 547.

15. Chang Po-Tuan and Liu I-Ming in Cleary, trans., *The Inner Teachings of Taoism,* 12.

16. Chang Po-Tuan and Liu I-Ming in Cleary, trans., *Taoist Classics,* vol. 2, 61.

17. Preservers of Truth sect from the Complete Reality school in Cleary, trans., *Taoist Classics,* vol. 2, 537.

18. Ibid., 538.

19. Chang Po-Tuan and Liu I-Ming in Cleary, trans., *The Inner Teachings of Taoism,* 45.

20. Wong, *Taoism: A Complete Introduction,* 183.

21. Korpiun, *Cranio-Sacral-Self-Waves,* 96.

22. Chang Po-Tuan and Liu I-Ming in Cleary, trans,. *The Inner Teachings of Taoism,* 45.

23. Ibid., 74.

24. Ge Hong in Campany, trans., *To Live as Long as Heaven and Earth.*

25. Chang Po-Tuan and Liu I-Ming in Cleary, trans., *The Inner Teachings of Taoism,* 46.

26. Ibid.

27. Kohn, *Introducing Daoism,* 104.

28. Robinet, *Taoism: Growth of a Religion,* 104.

29. Chang Po-Tuan and Liu I-Ming in Cleary, trans., *The Inner Teachings of Taoism,* 42.

30. Wong, *Taoism: An Essential Guide,* 175.

31. Chao Pi-Chen in Luk, trans., *Taoist Yoga,* 59.

32. Needham and Lu Gwei Dien, *Science and Civilisation in China,* vol. 5, part V, 121.

33. Chia, *Fusion of the Five Elements,* 4–5.

34. Chia, *Healing Light of the Tao,* 36–37.

35. Liu I-Ming in Cleary, trans., *The Inner Teachings of Taoism,* 52.

36. Ibid., 97.

37. Chang Po-Tuan and Liu I-Ming in Cleary, trans., *The Taoist Classics,* vol. 2, 46.

38. John of the Cross, *The Collected Works of St. John of the Cross.*

39. Liu I-Ming in Cleary, trans., *The Inner Teachings of Taoism,* 52.

40. Liu I-Ming in Cleary, trans., *I Ching.*

41. William Wei and Mantak Chia, www.universal-tao.com/article/supplementary.html.

42. Needham and Lu Gwei Dien, *Science and Civilisation in China,* vol. 5, part V, 66.

43. Chia, *Tan Tien Chi Kung,* 75.

44. Pregadio, *Great Clarity: Daoism and Alchemy,* 112.

45. Lu Dong-Pin in Wong, trans., *The Teachings of Immortals Chung and Lu,* 71–74.

46. Ibid., 82.

47. Robinet in Pregadio, ed., *The Encyclopedia of Taoism,* vol. 2, 862.

48. Rowan, *Subpersonalities.*

49. Holmes, *The Inner World Outside.*

50. Pregadio, *The Encyclopedia of Taoism,* vol. 1, 81.

51. Hussein in Pregadio, ed., *The Encyclopedia of Taoism,* vol. 1, 522–23.

52. Csikszentmihalyi in Pregadio, ed., *The Encyclopedia of Taoism,* vol. 1, 591. See also Chia, *The Taoist Soul Body.*

53. Robinet in Pregadio, ed., *The Encyclopedia of Taoism,* vol. 1, 210.

54. Ibid., 224.

55. Esposito in Pregadio, ed., *The Encyclopedia of Taoism,* vol. 2, 988.

56. Despeux in Pregadio, ed., *The Encyclopedia of Taoism,* vol. 2, 770.
57. Robinet in Pregadio, ed., *The Encyclopedia of Taoism,* vol. 1, 224.
58. Chang Po-Tuan and Liu I-Ming in Cleary, trans., *The Inner Teachings of Taoism,* 19.
59. Chia, www.universal-tao.com/special/kan_li.html.
60. Liu I-Ming in Cleary, trans., *The Inner Teachings of Taoism,* 25.
61. Lu Dong-Pin in Wilhelm, trans., *The Secrets of the Golden Flower,* 56.

## Chapter 4.
## Warm-Ups for Self-Practice

1. Kohn, *The Taoist Experience,* 167–68.
2. Ishida, "Body and Mind: The Chinese Perspective," 52.
3. *Lord Gold Tower's Scripture of the Three Prime and Perfect Ones,* in Kohn, trans., *Daoist Dietetics,* 127.
4. Lao-tzu in Wong, trans., *Cultivating Stillness,* 49.
5. Kohn, trans., *Daoist Dietetics,* 126.
6. Lao-tzu in Wong, trans., *Cultivating Stillness,* 49.
7. Kohn, trans., *Daoist Dietetics,* 124.
8. Lao-tzu in Wong, trans., *Cultivating Stillness,* 48–50.
9. Pregadio, *The Encyclopedia of Taoism,* vol. 1, 845.

## Chapter 5.
## The Greatest Kan and Li Formulas

1. Lu Dong-Pin in Wilhelm, trans., *The Secrets of the Golden Flower,* 33.
2. Ge Hong in Pregadio, "Early Daoist Meditation and the Origins of Inner Alchemy," 129; also see: www.goldenelixir.com/taoism/texts_baopu_zi.html.
3. Chang Po-Tuan and Liu I-Ming in Cleary, trans., *The Inner Teachings of Taoism,* 52.

## Chapter 6.
## Supplemental Practices

1. Preservers of Truth sect from the Complete Reality school in Cleary, trans., *The Taoist Classics,* vol. 2, 537.
2. Matthew 3:16, *King James Bible.*
3. Wong, *The Shambhala Guide to Taoism,* 183.
4. Chang Po-Tuan and Liu I-Ming in Cleary, trans., *The Inner Teachings of Taoism,* 74.
5. Lu Dong-Pin in Wong, trans., *The Teachings of Immortals Chung and Lu,* 9.
6. Wong, *The Shambhala Guide to Taoism,* 183.
7. Adapted from Colossians 1:16, *King James Bible:* "For by him were all things

created, that are in heaven, and that are in earth, visible and invisible, whether they be thrones, or dominions, or principalities, or powers: all things were created by him, and for him."

8. Chang Po-Tuan and Liu I-Ming in Cleary, trans., *The Inner Teachings of Taoism,* 45–46.
9. Pregadio, *The Encyclopedia of Taoism,* vol. 1, 797.
10. Lu Dong-Pin in Wong, trans., *The Teachings of Immortals Chung and Lu,* 96.
11. Lu Dong-Pin in Wilhem, trans., *The Secrets of the Golden Flower,* 73.

## Chapter 7.
## Diet for the Greatest Kan and Li Practice

1. "Highest Chi Scripture on Nourishing Life and Embryo Respiration" in Kohn, trans., *Daoist Dietetics,* 165.
2. Eisen, *Chinese Bigu,* http://yang-sheng.com/p=3874 (accessed October 15, 2011).
3. Jackowicz, "Ingestion, Digestion and Regestation: The Complexies of Absorption of Qi," 82.
4. Modena and Fieni, "Amniotic Fluid Dynamics," *Acta Bio Medica Ateneo Parmense* 75(1) (2004): 11.
5. Maciocia, *The Foundations of Chinese Medicine,* 45.
6. Kohn, trans., *Daoist Dietetics,* 165.
7. Stanley, Wynne, "Gastrointestinal Satiety Signals III," *American Journal of Physiology—Gastrointestinal Liver Physiology* 286: 693–97.
8. Eskildsen, *Ascetism in Early Taoist Religion,* 60–61.
9. Wood, "Practical Experience with Deathbringers," www.daoiststudies.org/dao/sites/default/files/Deathbringers_0.pdf, p8 (accessed December 2011).
10. Ibid., 12.
11. Guarner et al., *World Gastroenterology Organisation Practice Guideline: Probiotics and Prebiotics,* www.worldgastroenterology.org/assets/downloads/en/pdf/guidelines/19_probiotics_prebiotics.pdf, World Gastroenterology Organisation (assessed May 2008).
12. Ibid.
13. Sullivan and Nord, "Probiotics and Gastrointestinal Diseases." See also www.worldgastroenterology.org/assets/downloads/en/pdf/guidelines/19_probiotics_prebiotics.pdf, World Gastroenterology Organisation, 2008.
14. Hazarika and Pandey, "Traditional Phyto-Remedies For Worm Infestations of Two Important Tribal Communities of Assam, India," 32–39.
15. Adiswarananda, *Meditation & Its Practices,* 418.

16. Kohn, trans., *Daoist Dietetics,* 130.
17. Reid, *The Tao of Health, Sex and Longevity,* 132.
18. Mishori, Otubu, et al., "The Dangers of Colon Cleansing," 454–57.
19. *Huang Ting Jing (Nei Ching)* in Needham and Lu Gwei-Dien, *Science and Civilisation in China,* vol. 5, part V, 151.
20. Ibid., 150.
21. Yang Chen-Fu in Wile, trans., *Tai-chi Touchstones,* 1.
22. Bayat-Movahed and Shayeeteh, "Effects of Qigong Exercises on 3 Different Parameters of Human Saliva," *Chinese Journal of Integrative Medicine* 14(4) (2008): 262–66.
23. Eisen, "Scientific Qi Exploration, Part13c: Qigong and Immunity," *Yang Sheu* (blog), May 15, 2011, http://yang-sheng.com/?p=2063.
24. Pregadio, *The Encyclopedia of Taoism,* vol. 2, 698.
25. Huang, *The Primordial Breath,* 1987.
26. Wei Hua-Cun, a famous female Taoist in the Western Jin dynasty (265–317). See: www.chinaculture.org/gb/en_aboutchina/2003-09/24/content_24764.htm (accessed December 2011).
27. Teacher Tou in Needham and Lu Gwei-Djen, *Science and Civilisation in Ancient China,* vol. 5, part V, 120.
28. Eskildsen, *Ascetism in Early Taoist Religion,* 60–61.
29. Wood, "Practical Experience with Deathbringers," www.daoiststudies.org/dao/sites/default/files/Deathbringers_0.pdf (accessed December 2011), 8.
30. Kohn, trans., *Daoist Dieteics,* 159–62.
31. Ibid., 150–58.
32. Eskildsen, *Ascetism in Early Taoist Religion,* 43–68.
33. Penny, ed., *Daoism in History,* 131.
34. See: www.daowest-cultivation.com/daoism/taoist-classics/yellow-court-scripture.html (accessed December 2011).
35. *Huang Ting Jing (Nei Ching)* in Needham and Lu Gwei-Djen, *Science and Civilisation in Ancient China,* vol. 5, part V, 151.
36. Teacher Tou (13C), "Teacher Tou's Pointers for Restoration of the Primary Vitalities" in Needham and Lu Gwei-Djen, *Science and Civilisation in Ancient China,* vol. 5, part V, 120.
37. Needham, and Lu Gwei-Djen, *Science and Civilisation in Ancient China,* vol. 5, part V, 100.
38. Eskildsen, *Ascetism in Early Taoist Religion,* 43.
39. Palmer, *Qigong Fever,* 151.
40. Eskildsen, *Asseticism in Early Taoist Religion,* 44.

41. Kohn, trans., *Daoist Dietetics,* 117.

42. Ibid., 150–58.

43. Schipper, *The Taoist Body,* 169.

44. Ibid., 170.

45. In Kohn, trans., *Daoist Dietetics,* 159.

46. Pitchford, *Healing with Whole Foods,* 577.

47. Ibid., 584.

48. Eskildsen, *Ascetism in Early Taoist Religion,* 43–68.

49. Tuckahoe is a Chinese herb which interestingly is a diuretic and not used as a tonic. See: Chinese Herbs Home, Tuckahoe (Fu Ling), http://chinese.herbs .webs-sg.com/articles_26.html.

50. Eskildsen, *Ascetism in Early Taoist Religion,* 52

51. Ibid., 60–61.

52. Ibid., 59.

53. See: www.yinyanghouse.com/theory/herbalmedicine/suan_zao_ren_tcm_ herbal_database/ (accessed December 2011).

54. Eskildsen, *Ascetism in Early Taoist Religion,* 58.

55. Chang Po-Tuan and Liu I-Ming in Cleary, trans., *The Inner Teachings of Taoism,* 57.

56. U.S. Preventive Services Task Force (USPSTF). See: www .uspreventiveservicestaskforce.org/index.html (accessed December 2011).

57. Tony Robbins quoted in Bowden, *Telling It Like It Is,* 465.

58. Mosley and Spencer, *The Fast Diet.*

59. Harvie, Pegington, Mattson, et al., "The Effects of Intermittent or Continuous Energy Restriction on Weight Loss and Metabolic Disease Risk Markers," 714–27.

60. Harvie and Howell, "Energy Restriction and the Prevention of Breast Cancer," 263–75.

61. Kroeger, Klempel, Bhutani, et al., "Improvement in Coronary Heart Disease Risk Factors during an Intermittent Fasting/Calorie Restriction Regimen."

62. Teng, Shahar, Manaf, et al., "Improvement of Metabolic Parameters in Healthy Older Adult Men Following a Fasting Calorie Restriction Intervention," 607–14.

63. Michalsen, "Prolonged Fasting as a Method of Mood Enhancement in Chronic Pain Syndromes," 80–87.

64. Fond, Macgregor, Leboyer, and Michalsen, "Fasting in Mood Disorders: Neurobiology and Effectiveness," 253–58.

65. Kerndt, Naughton, Driscoll, and Loxtercamp, "Fasting: The History, Pathophysiology and Complications," 379.

66. Fond, Macgregor, Leboyer, and Michalsen, "Fasting in Mood Disorders: Neurobiology and Effectiveness," 253–58.

67. Ibid.

## Chapter 8.
## Home Practice: Embryo to Full Gestation

1. Liu I-Ming in Cleary, trans., *I Ching,* 174.

2. Ibid., 229.

3. Wong, *Taoism: A Complete Introduction,* 183.

4. Lu Dong-Pin in Wilhelm, trans., *The Secrets of the Golden Flower,* 51.

5. Liu I-Ming and Chang Po-Tuan in Cleary, trans., *The Inner Teachings of Taoism,* 97.

6. Liu I-Ming in Cleary, trans., *I Ching,* 17.

7. Li Dao-Chun in Cleary, *The Taoist Classics,* vol. 2, 355.

8. Liu I-Ming in Cleary, trans., *I Ching,*162.

9. Preservers of Truth sect from the Complete Reality school in Cleary, trans., *The Taoist Classics,* 536.

10. Wei Po-Yang, quoted by the Preservers of Truth sect in Cleary, trans., *The Taoist Classics*, 545.

11. Eskildsen, trans., "The Plain Dao of the Xiandao Jing," Sixth International Conference on Daoist Studies, Conference Paper (Los Angeles, 2010).

12. Chang Po-Tuan and Liu I-Ming in Cleary, trans., *The Taoist Classics,* 168.

13. Chang Po-Tuan and Liu I-Ming in Cleary, trans., *The Inner Teachings of Taoism,* 39.

14. Ibid., 38.

15. Lu Dong-Pin in Wilhelm, trans., *The Secrets of the Golden Flower.*

16. Liu I-Ming in Cleary, trans., *I Ching,* 229. Bracketed text added by the authors.

17. Lu Dong-Pin in Wilhelm, trans., *The Secrets of the Golden Flower,* 31.

18. Ibid., 63.

19. Eskildsen, *Ascetism in Early Taoist Religion,* 52.

20. Lu Dong-Pin in Wilhelm, trans., *The Secrets of the Golden Flower,* 5.

21. Ibid., 58.

## Glossary

1. Ge Hong, Bao Pu Tzu, quoted in Needham and Lu Gwei Djen, *Science and Civilisation in Ancient China,* vol. 5, part V, 143.

2. Pregadio, *Great Clarity: Daoism and Alchemy,* 207.

3. Ibid., 67.

4. Ibid., 69.

5.  Ibid., 210.

6.  Cleary, trans., *I Ching,* 25.

7.  Wong, trans., *The Teachings of Immortals Chung and Lu,* 95.

8.  Ibid., 100. See also Luk, *Taoist Yoga,* 210.

9.  Pregadio, *Great Clarity: Daoism and Alchemy,* 207.

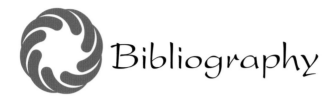
# Bibliography

Adiswarananda, Swami. *Meditation & Its Practices: A Definitive Guide to Techniques and Traditions of Meditation in Yoga and Vedanta.* Woodstock, Vt.: SkyLight Paths, 2007.

Bayat-Movahed, S., and Y. Shayeeteh "Effects of Qigong Exercises On 3 Different Parameters of Human Saliva." *Chinese Journal of Integrative Medicine* 14(4) (December 2008): 262–66.

Blake, William. *The Complete Poetry and Prose of William Blake.* Edited by David Erdman. Berkeley: University of California Press, 1982.

Bokenkamp, Stephen, ed. *Early Daoist Scriptures.* Berkeley: University of California Press, 1997.

Bowden, Paul. *Telling It Like It Is: A Book of Quotations.* Create Space Independent Publishing Platform, 2011.

Bushell, William, and Erin Olivia, eds. "Longevity Regeneration and Optimum Health Integrating Eastern and Western Perspectives." *Annals of the New York Academy of Science.* N.J.: Wiley, 2009.

Byrne, Patrick, trans. *Tao Te Ching: The Way of Virtue by Lao Tzu.* New York: Square One, 2002.

Campany, Robert, trans. *To Live as Long as Heaven and Earth: A Translation and Study of Ge Hong's Tradition of Divine Transcendents.* Berkeley: University of California Press, 2002.

Chao Pi Chen. "The Secrets of Cultivating Essential Nature and Eternal Life." In *The Sexual Teachings of the Ancient Chinese Masters,* translated by Lu Kuan-Yu. London: Rider, 1970.

Chang, Stephen T. *The Great Tao.* San Francisco: Tao Publishing, 1985.

Chen Chao-Hsiu, trans. *Tao Te Ching Cards.* London: Connections, 2003.

Chen Kai Guo and Shun Chao Zheng. *Opening the Dragon Gate: The Making of a Modern Taoist Wizard.* Translated by Thomas Cleary. Boston: Tuttle Publishing, 1996.

Chia, Mantak. *Fusion of the Five Elements.* Rochester, Vt.: Destiny Books, 2007.

———. *Golden Elixir Chi Kung.* Rochester, Vt.: Destiny Books, 2005.

———. *The Taoist Soul Body: Harnessing the Power of Kan and Li.* Rochester, Vt.: Destiny Books, 2007.

———. *Tan Tien Chi Kung: Foundational Exercises for Empty Force and Perineum Power.* Rochester, Vt.: Destiny Books, 2004.

Chia, Mantak, and Andrew Jan. *Tai Chi Wu Style.* Rochester, Vt.: Destiny Books, 2013.

Chia, Mantak, and Tao Huang. *Door to All Wonders: Application of the Tao Te Ching.* Chiang Mai, Thailand: Universal Tao Publications, 2001.

Cleary, Thomas, trans. *I Ching.* Boston: Shambhala, 1986.

———, trans. *Immortal Sisters: Secrets of Taoist Women.* Boston: Shambhala, 1989.

———, comp. and trans. *Taoist Meditation: Methods for Cultivating a Healthy Mind and Body.* Boston: Shambhala, 2000.

———. *Practical Taoism.* Boston: Shambhala, 1996.

———, trans. *The Inner Teachings of Taoism.* Boston: Shambhala, 2001.

———, trans. *The Taoist Classics: The Collected Translations,* vol. 1. Boston: Shambhala, 2003.

———, trans. *The Taoist Classics: The Collected Translations,* vol. 2. Boston: Shambhala, 2003.

Cooper, J. C. *Taoism: The Way of the Mystic.* North Hamptonshire, England: Aquarian Press, 1972.

———. "The Symbolism of the Taoist Garden." *Studies in Comparative Religion* 11(4) (Autumn 1977). Also available online: www.studiesincomparativereligion.com/uploads/ArticlePDFs/260.pdf.

Davis, Tenney L., and Chen Kuo-Fu. "Shang-Yang Tzu, Taoist Writer and Commentator on Alchemy." *Harvard Journal of Asiatic Studies* 7(2) (July 1942): 126–29.

Demasi, Franco. "The Paedophile and His Inner World: Theoretical and clinical Considerations on the Analysis of a Patient." *International Journal Psychoanalysis* 88 (2007): 147–65.

Eisen, Martin. "Scientific Qi Exploration, Part 13c: Qigong and Immunity," *Yang Shen* (blog), May 15, 2011, http://yang-sheng.com/?p=2063.

Emoto, Masaru. *The True Power of Water: Healing and Discovering Ourselves.* New York: Atria Books, an imprint of Simon and Schuster, 2005.

Eskildsen, Stephen. *Ascetism in Early Taoist Religion.* Albany, New York: State University of New York, 1998.

Esposito, Monica. "Longmen Taoism in Qing China: Doctrinal Ideal and Local Reality." *Journal of Chinese Religion* 29 (2001): 191–231.

Ettington, Martin K. *Immortality: A History and How To Guide: Or How to Live to 150 Years and Beyond.* Lexington, Ky.: mkettingtonbooks.com, 2008.

Feng, Gia, and Jane English, trans. *Tao de Ching*. New York: Vintage Books, Random House, 1972.

Fond, Guillaume, Alexandra Macgregor, Marion Leboyer, and Andreas Michalsen. "Fasting in Mood Disorders: Neurobiology and Effectiveness. A Review of the Literature." *Psychiatry Research* 209(3) (2013): 253–58.

Fung, Yu-Lan, trans. *Chuang Tzu: A New Selected Translation with an Exposition of the Philosophy of Kuo Hsiang*. Beijing: Foreign Language Press, 1989.

Girardot, Norman J. *Myth and Meaning in Early Taoism: The Theme of Chaos (Hun Tun)*. Berkeley: University of California Press, 1988.

Goethe, Johann Wolfgang von. *Faust: A Tragedy*. Translated by Bayard Taylor. Leipzig: Brockhaus, 1872.

Gulik, Robert H. van. *Sex Life in Ancient China: A Preliminary Survey of Chinese Sex and Society from ca 1500 BC till 1644 AD*. Leiden, Netherlands: E. J. Brill, 1961.

Hammer, Leon. *Dragon Rises, Red Bird Flies: Psychology and Chinese Medicine*. Wellingborough, England: Crucible, 1990.

Harvie, Michelle, and Anthony Howell. "Energy Restriction and the Prevention of Breast Cancer." *Proceedings of the Nutrition Society* 71(2) (2012): 263–75.

Harvie, Michelle N., Mary Pegington, Mark P. Mattson, et al. "The Effects of Intermittent or Continuous Energy Restriction on Weight Loss and Metabolic Disease Risk Markers: A Randomized Trial in Young Overweight Women." *International Journal of Obesity* 35(5) (2010): 714–27.

Hazarika, P., and B. K. Pandey. "Traditional Phyto-Remedies for Worm Infestations of Two Important Tribal Communities of Assam, India." *Asian Journal of Traditional Medicines* 5(1) (2010): 32–39.

He, Master. www.daowest-cultivation.com/taoism/taoist-classics/yellow-court-inner-view-scripture.html. Viewed online December 2011.

Holmes, Paul. *The Inner World Outside: Object Relations Theory and Psychodrama*. London: Routledge, 1992.

Huang, Jane, and Michael Wurmbrand. *The Primordial Breath: An Ancient Chinese Way of Prolonging Life through Breath Control. Volume 1: Seven Treatises from the Taoist Canon, the Tao Tsang*. Torrance, Calif.: Original Books, 1990.

Jackowicz, Stephen. "Ingestion, Digestion and Regestation: The Complexities of Absorption of Qi." In *Daoist Body Cultivation,* edited by Livia Kohn, 82. Magdalena, N.M.: Three Pines Press, 2006.

John of the Cross. *The Collected Works of St. John of the Cross*. Translated by Kieran Kavanaugh and Otilio Rodriguez. Washington: ICS Pub., 1973.

Katz, Steven. *Mysticism and Religious Traditions*. Oxford: Oxford University Press, 1983.

Kerndt, Peter R., James L. Naughton, Charles E. Driscoll, and David A. Loxtercamp.

"Fasting: The History, Pathophysiology and Complications." *Western Journal of Medicine* 137(5) (1982): 379.

Kohn, Livia, ed. *Daoist Body Cultivation*. Magdalena, N.M.: Three Pines Press, 2006.

———, trans. *Daoist Dietetics: Food for Immortality*. Dunedin, Fla.: Three Pines, 2010.

———. *Early Chinese Mysticism, Philosophy and Soteriology in the Taoist Tradition*. N. J.: Princeton University Press, 1992.

———. "Guarding the One." Chap. 5 in *Taoist Meditation and Longevity Techniques,* ed. Livia Kohn. Ann Arbor: University of Michigan Center for Chinese Studies, 1989.

———. *Introducing Daoism*. University Park, Pa.: Journal of Buddhist Ethics, 2009.

———, ed. *The Taoist Experience: An Anthology*. Albany: State University of New York Press, 1993.

———, ed. *Taoist Meditation and Longevity Techniques*. Michigan: University of Michigan Center for Chinese Studies, 1989.

———, trans. *Taoist Mystical Philosophy: The Scripture of Western Ascension*. Albany: State University of New York Press, 1991.

Kohn, Livia, and Robin Wang, eds. *Internal Alchemy*. Magdalena, N.M.: Three Pines Press, 2009.

Komjathy, Louis. *Cultivating Perfection: Mysticism and Self-Transformation in Early Quanzhen Daoism*. Leiden, Netherlands: Brill, 2007.

———. *Daoist Texts in Translation*. Excerpt posted at www.daoistcenter.org/advanced.html. Posted on September 15, 2003; updated on August 10, 2004.

Korpiun, Olaf J. *Cranio-Sacral-Self-Waves: A Scientific Approach to Cranio-Sacral Therapy*. Berkeley, Calif.: North Atlantic Books, 2011.

Kroeger, Cynthia M., Monica C. Klempel, Surabhi Bhutani, et al. "Improvement in Coronary Heart Disease Risk Factors during an Intermittent Fasting/Calorie Restriction Regimen: Relationship to Adipokine Modulations." *Nutrition & Metabolism* 9(98) (2012).

Kwok, Man Ho, trans. *Tao de Ching*. Brisbane: Element, 1993.

Li, Shi-Zhen, and F. P. Smith et al. *Chinese Medicinal Herbs: A Modern Edition of a Classic Sixteenth-Century Manual*. Mineola, N.Y.: Dover, 2003.

Loewe, Michael. *Chinese Ideas of Life and Death*. London: George Allan & Unwin, 1982.

———. *Ways to Paradise: The Chinese Quest for Immortality*. London: George Allan & Unwin, 1979.

Luk, Charles. *Taoist Yoga: The Sexual Teachings of the Ancient Chinese Masters*. London: Rider, 1970.

Maciocia, Giovanni. *The Foundations of Chinese Medicine: A Comprehensive Text for Acupuncturists and Herbalists.* Edinburgh: Churchill Livingstone, 1989.

Mah, Kenneth, and Yitzchak M. Binik. "The Nature of Human Orgasm: A Critical Review of Major Trends." *Clinical Psychology Review* 21(6) (2001): 823–56.

Michalsen, Andreas. "Prolonged Fasting as a Method of Mood Enhancement in Chronic Pain Syndromes: A Review of Clinical Evidence and Mechanisms." *Current Pain and Headache Reports* 14(2) (2010): 80–87.

Miller, James. *Chinese Religions in Contemporary Societies.* Santa Barbara, Calif.: ABC CLIO, 2006.

Mindich, Jeffrey. *Taiwan Review.* http://taiwanreview.nat.gov.tw/ct.asp?xItem= 107961&CtNode=, 09/01/2011. Viewed online December 2011.

Mishori, Ranit, Aye Otubu, et al. *The Journal of Family Practice* 60(8) (August 2011): 454–57.

Modena, Alberto Bacchi, and Stefania Fieni. "Amniotic Fluid Dynamics." *Acta Bio Medica Ateneo Parmense* 75(1) (2004): 11–13.

Mosley, Michael, and Mimi Spencer. *The Fast Diet: Lose Weight, Stay Healthy, and Live Longer with the Simple Secret of Intermittent Fasting.* London: Short Books, 2013.

Needham, Joseph, and Lu Gwei Dien. *Science and Civilisation in China: Volume 5, Chemistry and Chemical Technology, Part II, Spagyrical Discovery and Invention—Magisteries of Gold and Immortality.* London: Cambridge at the University Press, 1974.

Needham, Joseph, and Lu Gwei Dien. *Science and Civilisation in China, Volume 5, Chemistry and Chemical Technology, Part V, Spagyrical Discovery and Invention—Physiological Alchemy.* London: Cambridge at the University Press, 1983.

Olsen, Brad. *Modern Esoteric: Beyond Our Senses,* vol. 1. San Francisco: CCC Publishing, 2014.

Olson, Stuart Alve. *The Jade Emperor's Mind Seal Classic: The Taoist Guide to Health, Longevity, and Immortality.* Rochester, Vt.: Inner Traditions, 2003.

Ospina, Maria. *Meditation Practices for Health: State of the Research.* Edmonton, Canada: Diane, 2007.

Palmer, David A. *Qigong Fever: Body, Science, and Utopia in China.* New York: Columbia University Press, 2007.

Palmer, Martin. *The Jesus Sutras: Recovering the Lost Religion of Taoist Christianity.* London: Judy Piatkus, 2001.

Penny, Benjamin, ed. *Daoism in History: Essays in Honour of Liu Tsun-Yan.* New York: Routledge, 2006.

Pregadio, Fabrizio. *9 Taoist Books on the Elixir: A Short Bibliography.* Mountain View, Calif.: Golden Elixir Press, 2009.

———. *Great Clarity: Daoism and Alchemy in Early Medieval China.* Stanford, Calif.: SUP, 2009.

———. *The Encyclopedia of Taoism,* vols. 1 and 2. New York: Routledge, 2007.

Pitchford, Paul. *Healing with Whole Foods: Oriental Traditions and Modern Nutrition.* Berkeley, Calif.: North Atlantic Books, 1993.

Reid, Daniel. *The Tao of Health, Sex, and Longevity.* London: Simon and Schuster, 2011.

Robinet, Isabelle. "Metamorphosis and Deliverance from the Corpse in Taoism." *History of Religions* 19(1) (August 1979): 37–70.

———. *Taoist Meditation: The Mao Shan Tradition of Great Purity.* Translated by Julian Pas and Norman Girardot. Albany, N.Y.: State University of New York Press, 1993.

———. *Taoism: Growth of a Religion.* Translated by Phyllis Brooks. Stanford, Calif.: Stanford University Press, 1997.

Rogers, Carol, and Linda K. Larkey et al. "A Review of Clinical Trials of Tai Chi and Qigong in Older Adults." *Western Journal of Nursing Research* 31(2) (March 2009): 245–79.

Rowan, John. *Subpersonalities: The People Inside Us.* London: Routledge, 1990.

Ruan Fang-Fu. *Sex in China: Studies in Sexology in Chinese Culture.* New York: Plenum, 1991.

Schipper, Kristofer. *The Taoist Body.* Translated by Karen Duval. Berkeley: University of California Press, 1993.

Stanley, Sarah, Katie Wynne, et al. "Gastrointestinal Satiety Signals III. Glucagon-Like Peptide 1, Oxyntomodulin, Peptide YY, and Pancreatic Polypeptide." *American Journal of Physiology—Gastrointestinal and Liver Physiology* 286 (May 2004): 693–97.

Steiner, Rudolf. *The Philosophy of Freedom: The Basis of a Modern World Conception.* Translated by Michael Wilson. London: Rudolph Steiner Press, 1999.

Sullivan, A., and C. E. Nord. "Probiotics and Gastrointestinal Diseases." *Journal of Internal Medicine* 257 (2005): 78–92.

Szekely, Edmond Bordeaux. "Fasting." *The Nazarene Way,* www.thenazareneway .com/diet/fasting.htm. Viewed online December 2011.

Teng, Nur Islami Mohd Fahmi, Suzana Shahar, Zahara Abdul Manaf, et al. "Improvement of Metabolic Parameters in Healthy Older Adult Men Following a Fasting Calorie Restriction Intervention." *Pakistan Journal of Nutrition* 12(7) (2013): 607–14.

Tierra, Michael. *The Way of Herbs.* New York: Simon and Schuster, 1998.

Wei, Hua-Cun. *Scripture of the Yellow Court* (Huang ting jing). www.chinaculture.org/ gb/en_aboutchina/2003-09/24/content_24764.htm. Viewed online December 2011.

Wilhelm, Richard, trans. *The Secrets of the Golden Flower: A Chinese Book of Life.* London: Routledge & Kegan Paul, 1975.

Wile, Douglas, trans. *T'ai-chi Touchstones: Yang Family Secret Transmissions.* Brooklyn, N.Y.: Sweet Chi Press, 2010.

———, trans. *Lost Tai-Chi Classics from the Late Ching Dynasty.* Albany: State University of New York Press, 1996.

Williams, C., and Terrence Barlow. *Chinese Symbolism and Art Motifs: A Comprehensive Handbook on Symbolism in Chinese Art through the Ages.* North Clarendon, Vt.: Tuttle, 1988.

Winn, Michael. "Daoist Internal Alchemy in the West." In *Internal Alchemy,* ed. Livia Kohn and Robin Wang. Magdalena, N.M.: Three Pines Press, 2009.

———. "Daoist Methods for Dissolving the Heart Mind." *Journal of Daoist Studies* 2 (2009): 177–84.

Wittgenstein, Ludwig. *Tractatus Logico-Philosophicus 6.431.* Viewed online January 2012: www.kfs.org/~jonathan/witt/t6431en.html.

Wood, J. Michael. "Practical Experience with Deathbringers." www.daoiststudies.org/dao/sites/default/files/Deathbringers_0.pdf. Viewed online December 2011.

Wong, Eva, trans. *Cultivating Stillness: A Taoist Manual for Transforming Body and Mind.* Boston: Shambhala, 1992.

———, trans. *Cultivating the Energy of Life: A Translation of the Hui-Ming Ching and its Commmentaries.* Boston: Shambhala, 1998.

———, trans. *Harmonizing Yin and Yang—A Manual of Taoist Yoga, Internal, External and Sexual: The Dragon and Tiger Classic.* Boston: Shambhala, 1997.

———, trans. *Nourishing the Essence of Life: The Outer, Inner, and Secret Teachings of Taoism.* Boston: Shambhala, 2004.

———. *Taoism: A Complete Introduction to the History, Philosophy and Practice of an Ancient Spiritual Tradition.* Boston: Shambhala, 1997.

———. *Taoism: An Essential Guide.* Boston: Shambhala, 2011.

———, trans. *The Teachings of Immortals Chung and Lu: The Tao of Health and Longevity, and Immortality.* Boston: Shambhala, 2000.

———. *Teachings of the Tao.* Boston: Shambhala, 1997.

World Gastroenterology Organisation. "Probiotics and Prebiotics." www.worldgastroenterology.org/assets/downloads/en/pdf/guidelines/19_probiotics_prebiotics.pdf, 2008. Viewed online December 2011.

Wu Lu-Chiang, and Tenney L. Davis, trans. "An Ancient Chinese Treatise on Alchemy Entitled Ts'an T'ung Ch'I." *Isis* 18(2) (October 1932): 210–89.

Yogananda, Paramahansa. *Autobiography of a Yogi.* Kolkata: Yogoda Satsanga Society of India, 2005.

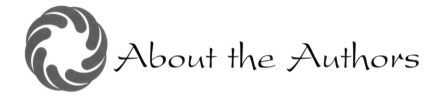

# About the Authors

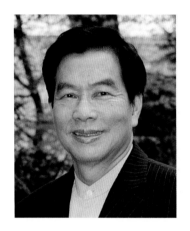

## MANTAK CHIA

Mantak Chia has been studying the Taoist approach to life since childhood. His mastery of this ancient knowledge, enhanced by his study of other disciplines, has resulted in the development of the Universal Healing Tao system, which is now being taught throughout the world.

Mantak Chia was born in Thailand to Chinese parents in 1944. When he was six years old, he learned from Buddhist monks how to sit and "still the mind." While in grammar school he learned traditional Thai boxing, and he soon went on to acquire considerable skill in aikido, yoga, and Tai Chi. His studies of the Taoist way of life began in earnest when he was a student in Hong Kong, ultimately leading to his mastery of a wide variety of esoteric disciplines, with the guidance of several masters, including Master I Yun, Master Meugi, Master Cheng Yao Lun, and Master Pan Yu. To better understand the mechanisms behind healing energy, he also studied Western anatomy and medical sciences.

Master Chia has taught his system of healing and energizing practices to tens of thousands of students and trained more than two thousand instructors and practitioners throughout the world. He has established centers for Taoist study and training in many countries around the globe. In June of 1990, he was honored by the International Congress of

Chinese Medicine and Qi Gong (Chi Kung), which named him the Qi Gong Master of the Year.

# ANDREW JAN

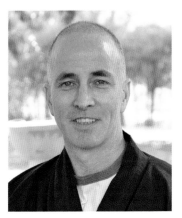

Dr. Andrew Jan is a senior instructor for the Universal Healing Tao system. He first became an instructor in 1992 and has been a senior instructor since 2001. He began studying martial arts as a young child, and has been studying the internal arts of Wu Shu for twenty-five years. His teachers include: Chen Lu, John Yuen (Blackburn Tai Chi Academy), Liu De-Ming (Associate Professor Martial Arts, Fujien University), Liu Hong-Chi (Beijing), Huo Dong-Li (Senior Judge, Beijing Wu Shu Federation), Zhu Tian-Cai (one of the contemporary "tigers" of Chen Jia Guo), and of course Master Mantak Chia.

Dr. Andrew Jan has won multiple medals in Push Hands competitions and a Full-Contact All Styles Lightweight Division in 1984 in Victoria. In 2000, he became the National Tai Chi and Wu Shu Champion in the over-forty section and also won first place in Wu Style, Yang Style, and Weapon divisions. He first studied Kan and Li in 1990 and has been teaching this practice since 2003.

Dr. Andrew Jan is currently practicing as an emergency medicine physician and medical acupuncturist. He also runs a private medical practice where he integrates Chinese and Western Medicine. He has a bachelor's degree in the arts as well as a master's degree in philosophy.

Dr. Andrew Jan was born in Australia to a Chinese father and an English mother. He has always found himself exploring and synthesizing Eastern and Western traditions, an ability he applies to healing as well as martial arts. He has to date coauthored four books with Mantak Chia on Tai Chi and advanced Taoist meditation. He is married to his loving wife and fellow practitioner, Fiona, with one daughter, Nikita.

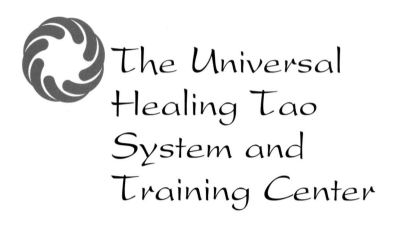

# The Universal Healing Tao System and Training Center

## THE UNIVERSAL TAO SYSTEM

The ultimate goal of Taoist practice is to transcend physical boundaries through the development of the soul and the spirit within the human. That is also the guiding principle behind the Universal Tao, a practical system of self-development that enables individuals to complete the harmonious evolution of their physical, mental, and spiritual bodies. Through a series of ancient Chinese meditative and internal energy exercises, the practitioner learns to increase physical energy, release tension, improve health, practice self-defense, and gain the ability to heal him- or herself and others. In the process of creating a solid foundation of health and well-being in the physical body, the practitioner also creates the basis for developing his or her spiritual potential by learning to tap in to the natural energies of the sun, moon, earth, stars, and other environmental forces.

The Universal Tao practices are derived from ancient techniques rooted in the processes of nature. They have been gathered and integrated into a coherent, accessible system for well-being that works directly with the life force, or chi, that flows through the meridian system of the body.

Master Chia has spent years developing and perfecting techniques for teaching these traditional practices to students around the world through ongoing classes, workshops, private instruction, and healing sessions, as well as books and video and audio products. Further information can be obtained at www.universal-tao.com.

## THE UNIVERSAL TAO TRAINING CENTER

The Tao Garden Resort and Training Center in northern Thailand is the home of Master Chia and serves as the worldwide headquarters for Universal Tao activities. This integrated wellness, holistic health, and training center is situated on eighty acres surrounded by the beautiful Himalayan foothills near the historic walled city of Chiang Mai. The serene setting includes flower and herb gardens ideal for meditation, open-air pavilions for practicing Chi Kung, and a health and fitness spa.

The center offers classes year round, as well as summer and winter retreats. It can accommodate two hundred students, and group leasing can be arranged. For information worldwide on courses, books, products, and other resources, see below.

## RESOURCES

Universal Healing Tao Center
274 Moo 7, Luang Nua, Doi Saket, Chiang Mai, 50220
    Thailand
Tel: (66)(53) 495-596 Fax: (66)(53) 495-852
E-mail: universaltao@universal-tao.com
Web site: www.universal-tao.com

For information on retreats and the health spa, contact:
Tao Garden Health Spa & Resort
E-mail: info@tao-garden.com, taogarden@hotmail.com
Web site: www.tao-garden.com

**Good Chi • Good Heart • Good Intention**

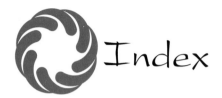<br>
**Index**

Page numbers in *italics* refer to illustrations.